HOW TO TAKE CARE OF YOU . . .

So You Can Take Care of OTHERS.

by

Sue Vineyard

Heritage Arts Publishing
1807 Prairie Avenue
Downers Grove, IL 60515
(312) 964-0841

Heritage Arts Publishing
1807 Prairie Avenue
Downers Grove, IL 60515
© 1987. Sue Vineyard
ISBN Number: #0-911029-06-0

Other Books by the Author:

Finding Your Way Through The Maze of Volunteer Management, 1981
Beyond Banquets Plaques and Pins, 1982
Fundraising for Hospices & Other Organizations, 1983
Marketing Magic for Volunteer Programs, 1984
101 Ideas for Volunteer Programs, 1986
101 Ways to Raise Resources, 1987

TABLE OF CONTENTS

Dedicated to all the Soul Mates in my life:

Wes, Bill, Bob and Meghan

Skrewe U.

s2

The Most Worthy Past Grand Matron

The Other Mother Superior

"K"

A Hawaiian Alligator

and

an incredible medical team:

Dr. Philip Hunter

Dr. Bruce Dillon

Jean Parker, RN/Ostomy Specialist

Arlana Jaros, RN

ACKNOWLEDGEMENTS

Grateful thanks to everyone who encouraged me as I wrote this very different type of book. After 6 technical, "management-style" texts, it was a new experience and took a lot of "sure you can" statements from close associates who insist it's a most needed work.

Special thanks to Mary Ann Lawson who watched out for grammar, punctuation and spelling goofs between her personal "ah-has's!"; Marlene Wilson who used her normal scalpel as she examined every word and phrase, thereby improving it vastly; to Richard Krajeski who, from his vantage as a trainer in caregiving, shared content suggestions; Elaine Yarbrough, who read it and played "cheerleader" and wise suggestor, and Jean Parker, RN, who kept yelling "RIGHT ON!" after looking at it's message. Also Great love and appreciation to Betty Mitchell who struggled to read my scrawl and transfer it into the language of the Apple.

I thank you all.

PROLOGUE

It happened swiftly. A sharp pain, then cramping that built to a crescendo that was beyond tolerance or belief.

Part of me was startled, shocked even, at the pain. Another, more honest part of me, said quietly, "You must have seen it coming. The signs were there for years."

Frustration set in as I convinced myself that I was experiencing yet another attack of diverticulitis. Calls to the doctor and the familiar advice to go to clear liquids and take the medicine I carried with me at all times followed during the first few hours after the onslaught of the attack.

As time passed and the pain increased, despite all efforts to reduce it, my frustration was slowly replaced by fear and a supressed conviction that something was terribly wrong . . . something beyond an inflamed colon that had plagued me for decades and seemed to have worsened dramatically during the past three years.

Doctors along the way had ascribed my concern over "stomach problems" to various life-stages: "Young mothers always have stomach problems", "You're just tense", "You may be going into early monopause."

When real problems such as blood in the stool emerged, the probable cause was shifted to "stress" with the ever popular Valium prescribed. In recent years several new doctors began to question my hectic life style as the possible culprit.

I chose to ignore their questions and apply temporary bandages, such as a few days of rest, convincing myself that I was taking care of "me". I rejected any suggestions that I slow down and stood firm on my refusal to take Valium or any equivalent. Instead I opted for yet another slug of Pepto Bismo or Milk of Magnesia and kept up my hectic schedule.

As I look back, I see that my "schdule" was more of a rat race than anything! Approximately 40-44 weeks out of the year I could be found racing for airplanes, sleeping in motels or dormitories, gulping down airport hotdogs, banquet creamed chicken, or restaurant offerings while I trained or keynoted conferences for volunteer managers across North America.

A typical day for me was being roused by a motel wake up call, grabbing a piece of toast and cup of tea in the lobby restaurant, being driven to a conference center by a stranger assigned to "host" me, speaking before an audience of up to 1500 for 6-8 hours with my only "breathers" being coffee breaks and lunch, where inevitably, someone would want to "pick my brain." The day would end with a madcap race for a plane, an exhausted ride home through the clouds, complete with a diet coke, a bag of peanuts and some rather indistinguishable meal served in a plastic container.

Days at home were full of desk work to catch up on the mounds of mail that accumulated during my travels, orders for any of my five books, calls requesting my training services up to two years in advance, and a mounting number of people seeking advice, counsel, and assistance with some challenge or problem. Between these demands I worked on writing books, a newsletter, and articles.

In short, I was systematically giving hunks of "me" to everyone else, with little thought about what might happen if I gave everything away.

Personal stress at home coincided with the natural stress of my work, but still I ignored its possible consequences.

I convinced myself that I was taking enough time for myself between trips; that I knew enough about stress control that I wouldn't allow real problems to take hold; that what I was doing for others was so important and so needed that risking and stretching were called for, and of course, that I wouldn't get caught by anything so seriously dangerous that I couldn't handle it.

I was wrong on all counts.

As the pain increased that July 4th of 1986, the reality of my situation refused to be denied. At 3 a.m. on the 5th, after 14 hours of increasingly excruciating pain, I went to the emergency room of the hospital. With my husband practically carrying me, I checked in to what was to be a long stay.

A quick examination by the attending physician produced a bevy of medical personnel, obviously concerned and trying to reassure me they would stop the pain as soon as the surgeon could get to the hospital and examine me. His appearance and learned assessment of the situation brought me the first realistic look at what had happened ... a ruptured colon and severe peritinitis, demanding immediate surgery to remove the involved colon area and create a colostomy.

When I awoke after surgery, I was surrounded by caring and concerned medical personnel of every variety, family that had been hastily summoned and wore a collective shade of grey on their faces, and a bevy of beeping, whirring and sucking machines that invaded every normal opening in my body and several newly created ones.

For three days people seemed to hover, reassuring me through stiff smiles that I was going to be alright. The phone was placed at my ear so that my closest friend, some 900 miles away, could join in the "hang in there" symphony. Other soulmates, frustrated at being miles distant in Washington, D.C., Colorado, North Carolina, and Minnesota, called to encourage my recovery, and my room began to look like a floral shop as well-wishers sent their love.

Improvement was measured in strange ways ... the removal of a machine or tube; sitting up; standing; my first three steps in the room (cause for a celebration by the staff and myself!) and my first venture into the hall for my initial real "walk", 22 steps, followed by a chorus of hurrahs!

Setbacks of resistance to colostomy applicances, sensitivity to surgical tape and two incidents of heart irregularity were outweighed by a gradual strengthening and the loving support and guidance of caring staff.

Through all this, my subsequent return home to convalesce for 3½ months and the planning of a return trip to the hospital to hopefully close the colostomy and do additional surgery on the colon brought on a million questions.

How had I, who admonished others to "take care of yourself, so that you can take care of others," come to the point of near death through stress related illness without seeing the warning signs of real trouble?

What steps could I have taken along my life's journey that could have produced different, healthier results?

And finally ... what could I gain from this experience that could not only prevent further problems for myself, but could also be shared with others in the hope of helping them prevent such a disaster?

This book is the answer.

More than a personal examination of what brought me to the operating table on that hot July night (although it does that by the nature of pointing out ignored stress points), I hope it will be a roadmap for the reader to assess and respond to the stressors that surround us everyday. It is written especially for the caregivers and helping professionals of our world, who like myself, dedicate their energies to caring for and about others in need, although it can be read and used by anyone who feels themselves giving more away than they are being given in return.

In addition to the words expressed, it is hoped that the tools found on these pages can be helpful as you proceed on your journey through life . . . dealing with the circumstances that surround you in a healthy and positive manner.

INTRODUCTION

Social workers, volunteers, teachers, nurses, clergy, doctors, lay leaders, volunteer directors, workers and leaders in government, clubs, charities, agencies, humanities, justice, the arts, recreation, health, etc. etc . . . .

All of the above and many more with related responsibilities frequently have two things in common:

1. They spend their energies and time serving
   or caring for others.
2. They have little energy or time left over
   for themselves.

Of the more than 10,000 people with whom I interact annually as a trainer, consultant and author, all of them are in the business of caring for others, either directly or indirectly.

As I travel I hear story after story of miracles they are bringing about for the good of others.

Unfortunately, I also hear many stories of stress, burnout, grief, exhaustion and illness from these same caregivers as they describe the toll their caring has taken on themselves personally.

As I look at my own story I now recognize in hindsight a similar pattern of giving so much away that too little reserve was left for my own personal wellness. I am almost (but not quite!) amused at recalling my fervent pleas to my audiences to "take care of yourself, because if you don't, how can you take care of others?"

Obviously I gave advice I ignored myself.

As caregivers we seem to fall into patterns of heeding the cries for help from clients, co-workers, patients, students, subordinates, members of the general public while at the same time ignoring or minimizing our own needs.

We frequently characterize our feelings by saying "everyone wants a hunk of me" or "I don't have anymore to give!" or "I'm pulled in 1,000 directions at once" and yet we go on giving and giving and giving.

After long hours at the office we often return home to families and friends who seek our help and guidance because we have built up a reputation for caring, compassion and the abilities to help. There seems to be no "time off".

We fall into a conviction that every wrong can and should be righted, every ill cured and every problem fixed . . . usually by us!

We fill our calendars with meetings and plans and appointments around our regular work schedule to such a point that only infrequently (if ever) do we leave time just for ourselves.

We look at time off as non-productive and we are often ill at ease when we have "nothing" to do.

Sadly after such a pattern becomes entrenched, we begin to experience symptoms of restlessness, dissatisfaction, and even resentment. We experience feelings of being overwhelmed, over-extended and exhausted. Headaches, muscle spasms, stomach problems and assorted aches and pains become commonplace though frequently ignored.

As negative feelings creep into our thoughts, they are immediately pushed back by guilt, "shoulds" and "oughts", and a psychological tug of war is begun that drains us all the more.

Our ability to think quickly and clearly begins to dull. Details escape us. Short term memory becomes a problem and juggling myriad details simultaneously becomes more and more difficult.

Spririts ebb. Joy is absent. Fun is nonexistent. Laughter is forced. Loneliness engulfs us. Self doubt and unanswerable questions haunt us. "Is it worth it?" "Does what I do really make a difference?" "Does anyone care?"

All of these symptoms, as they affect our physical, emotional, mental and spiritual dimensions, are those typical to the caregivers of the world.

As we look at the enormous responsibilities we have for the well-being, nurturing, lives and growth of others, our own needs slip to the background, labeled incorrectly (and dangerously) as being at least "lesser" and at the extreme, "insignificant".

We must readjust our thinking and retrain our instincts so that as we assess our responsibilities, we place ourselves among our top priorities.

We must assess how we are and take steps towards our own wellness before we try to bring about wellness in others.

We must wash away feelings of guilt about caring for ourselves and replace them with a conviction that our own well being is the best help we can offer others.

10

We need to understand that when we have a good relationship with our physical, mental, emotional and spiritual dimensions; when we have a sound support system; when we build in time to play, laugh, love and enjoy, we THEN will have the personal resources to serve others in whatever ways are necessary.

Such a pattern will go a long way to ward off the burnout, illness, stress, grief and uncreative thinking that can lead to leaving the field of human service and thus those who need us so desperately.

And that is the ultimate goal.

To help ourselves so we can help others.

It is to this end that this book is written . . . as a roadmap or even a survival guide for people who give their energies in service to others. It is written in the fondest hope that it will guide the readers to a more balanced, healthful wellness which can equip them to be even more effective in positively impacting the lives of others.

After all, if we don't take care of ourselves, how can we take care of others?

CHAPTER I

CHANGE

ACCEPTING CHANGE ... OR: "HAVE BAG, WILL TRAVEL"...

The biggest change I've ever had to face in my life was adjusting to a colostomy.

In trying to help me adjust during those first days after the surgery, several people described it to me as a "nuisance."

The word is far too weak for the reality of it.

Never before have I been more conscious of how one change can affect you physically, mentally, emotionally, and spiritually.

First came the physical adjustment . . . to a new body image; feelings of vulnerability and the constant care of an appliance that was completely foreign. Suddenly I found myself having to be aware of all the various "parts" . . . wafer, bag, clip, stoma paste, flange, etc. . . . and the concern that everything would work as it should. Odor became almost an obsession with me, and I quickly experimented with every perfume and deodorizer I could get my hands on! Unpredictability topped off my worry list, and for the first time in my life I had to surrender any notion of total control over my life.

Emotionally I experienced an almost immeasurable effect as I felt "different" and changed deeply, without being able to define exactly how. I was plagued with questions about my ability to continue on with my career as it had been for seven years . . . traveling, training, and speaking before large audiences. An offshoot of this concern became my search for proper clothing that would not "reveal" anything, and my need for assurance from those closest to me that indeed, everything looked normal.

I also had to deal with a deeper consideration of how tentative life really is. Having come within a hair's breath of the great lecture hall in the sky made me think more deeply about how I was spending my time and energes and about the priorities in my life. All this made me impatient with conversations that focused on short range thinking or what I now considered to be petty considerations.

Mentally I found that the colostomy and its safety were never off my mind. I had been used to being able to block anything I wished from my thoughts as I concentrated on what I was doing . . . writing, training, etc. Now, I could no longer do that, and I felt anger and frustration at the loss of this ability.

Spiritually I found myself digging deeper into the spiritual quality of my life, including an estrangement from my organized church and a frustration with what I considered to be a focus by churches on institutionalization rather than the business of caring for people and their needs. My own walk with God came under careful scrutiny as I reached down for strength and compassion.

All of these considerations and impacts came tumbling down on me at the same time, and all of them brought me to a fascination with change. As I dealt with the changes that were happening to me after the surgery, I began to realize that many major changes had happened in my past, but I had not really considered their impact on me.

The more I thought about change, the more I realized how frequently I, and the many helping professionals around me, must deal with change as it relates to others, but almost never really assess the effect those same changes have on us.

In retrospect I realized that had I paid more attention to the changes in my life over the past three years, I would have more clearly been aware of the mounting stress and possibly saved myself from such physical damage.

In one three month period, for instance, my eldest son was married and separated, my husband had a heart attack, my house flooded, my younger son was in an accident that totaled the family car, my mother had a stroke, and my father had cancer surgery. During all this, I continued on with my work, projecting to my audiences that "all was well."

I am not suggesting that such monumental changes must occur before you have problems . . . it takes far fewer to cause stress to take its toll. I do hope, however, that you look closely at change, to assess its impact on you physically, mentally, emotionally, relationally, and spiritually. Such an assessment may save your life!

CATEGORIES OF CHANGE . . .

A good place to start in your personal quest to take better care of yourself is an honest appraisal of the changes that have occurred in your life.

As you begin to examine the changes that affect you, consider the following categories as critical aspects of a wholistically healthy you:

1. Personal or business relationships
2. Changes in home life
3. Personal changes (illness, success, habits, lifestyle, etc.)
4. Work and financial changes
5. Inner changes (spiritual, social or political awareness, self-image, values, dreams, etc.)
6. Changes that effect people you seek to serve
7. Changes that effect people with whom you are close

Had I been watching what was really going on inside of me I would have seen that changes were occurring in all seven categories at once . . . a real danger signal!

Change is all around and in us. It is often said that the only thing that will never change is the existence of change.

Our challenge is to meet change with awareness and adaptability, assessing its impact on us personally and balancing this impact with healing acceptance and a commitment to self-care during the natural transitions that occur.

ASSESSING CHANGE . . .

Everyone encounters changes in their lives, from lesser ones (new neighbors, co-workers, etc.) to major ones (loss of a spouse, job, or health). The trick seems to be to accurately assess the effect these changes have on you while also trying to positively adjust to them so they do not produce unnecessary and negative stress.

Please note that I point to the dangers of negative stress as a distinction between stress that is good and stress that is bad. Often we brand all stress as "bad," and this is simply not true.

In our work to help others, we encounter many stressful times . . . when we are getting a new program off the ground, when we discover a challenge, when we must find alternative ways to accomplish our goals . . . and these times produce the adrenelin we need to make things happen. This is positive stress. How frequently we say of someone, "they certainly rose to the occasion" and in so saying are really referring to someone who encountered stress (usually though change) and found ways to adapt and find a positive solution to the challenge.

Thomas Holmes and Richard Rahe have created a rather famous Social Readjustment Rating Scale[1] that is familiar to most of us. It lists a number of life events and we are asked to check those that have occurred in our life in the previous year. Each is given a numerical weight and the score of the combined numbers seems to indicate whether or not the test taker will experience any physical problems in the near future.

I have included their test on page 35 for you to take, and I urge you to do so as you assess the impact that changes during the past year may have on your physical health.

In addition to their test I have created a broader list of life occurrences you may have encountered during the last year which I have included on page 37 of this book.

It shows different categories of your life for you to assess so that you might begin to have a broader perspective of changes as they effect your well-being. You can rate each event as positive, negative, or neutral and also indicate when the change occurred in order to measure times of particular stress.

There is no fancy scoring at its conclusion. Only you can measure the cumulative weight of the changes in your life. My Life Events Check List is simply an assessment tool to bring the changes into focus so that you may become aware of them as you assess what is truly going on inside of yourself.

I truly believe that had I had such a list before my surgery, to assess the stress I was under, I would have been better equipped to avert the disaster of the colostomy and the disintegration of my own health.

CUMULATIVE EFFECT OF CHANGES . . .

In 1981 I wrote my first book, Finding Your Way Through The Maze Of Volunteer Management.[2]

It was an 8½ by 11, 72 page work weighing less than 6 ounces, and therefore taking up little space on a bookshelf.

Imagine my surprise when it took three strong men and one fair sized truck to deliver my first order of 3000 of these "little" books. Their cumulative boxes spilled out of the storage space I had set aside and into an adjacent hallway!

Obviously, I had not calculated what this number of books would look like and therefore, had not planned well enough for their impact.

The same is true for cumulative changes and/or stress.

A friend moves, your favorite store closes, your youngest child goes off to school, the board requires a new reporting system, and your office is rearranged.

None of these occurrences is lifeshattering. None, by themselves, is overwhelming. There is, however, a collective weight as each brings about a demand for change, and a readjustment of your "normal" (and therefore familiar) way of life.

It is critical that we look at cumulative change and assess resultant stress. A layering of small changes can add up to continued uncertainty and a feeling of being "off balance" and therefore take on added significance to our health, well-being, and effectiveness.

Go back and look at your Life Events Assessment. For those changes you marked as either positive or negative, how many were clustered in a short time span or occurred at exactly the same time?

Were there any that came so close together that you buried your feelings about some changes so you could concentrate on other, more demanding ones? This could be a clue to uncovering some unresolved stress, grief, or frustration.

When, in the space of a few weeks, my husband suffered his heart attack, one son was in an auto accident, and both parents had sudden, serious health problems, my older son and his new bride separated.

Although I recognized this as a major disappointment and concern, I shoved it to the back of my mind, concentrating on the health of my family members instead.

It was not until one year later that circumstances made me realize that the grief of the loss of my daughter-in-law with whom I was very close, had never really been acknowledged or resolved. Instead, it had been buried and ignored, causing an unresolved grief that was "stuck" in an unproductive and stress-creating phase.

It is not unusual to bury one or more stressors subconsciously when too many occur at once. We become healthier when we can uncover our buried stress, recognizing its impact and come to grips with our feelings, so that we can move on to coping mechanisms.

Frequently in consulting with organizations, I find that problems with staff, efficiency, relationships, etc. come about at the time of accumulated changes in the workings of that organization.

One charity complained of lack of cooperation and great resistance to a new organizational structure imposed by the national leadership. Upon investigation, I found that at the same time that the new structure was to take effect, the group had moved to a new headquarters, the staff had to adjust to open-concept office space, a new Regional Director was brought in, a favorite adminstrator had been demoted, and all new reporting systems had been inaugurated. No wonder there was stress and resistance ... these were simply too many changes coming at once!

A major factor in the climate of an organization is the sum of the feelings held by the people involved and the changes imposed at any given time. The more that the changes are imposed rather than chosen, the more that resistance will result. When these changes come in rapid-fire succession, or even at the exact same time, we have a cumulative stress factor in our lives.

It is critical that we each look at the life events and changes that are happening at any one period of time. Each change needs to be observed from the angle of its effect on us and resultant feelings that need to be aired and examined rather than suppressed. My dear friend and soul mate, Elaine Yarbrough who holds a PhD in Communication and teaches conflict management around the nation, cautions us to understand that feelings are facts.

We must examine the facts of our feelings as we encounter change, so that we can assess their impact, with the goal of taking necessary steps to positively counteract any negative signals they are sending to our bodies, our minds, and most importantly, our souls.

I urge you to take time now to think through any major changes that have occurred in your life in the past three years which may have been "buried" due to the need to deal with other matters. Can you examine the feelings you had about those changes? Are there any responses that are unresolved?

Take a good look deep inside of you and clean house of those that may have piled up in a corner of your heart at a particularly stressful time!

CHANGES THAT SURROUND US ...

In William Bridge's book, Transitions, he quotes futurist Alvin Toffler: "Change is avalanching upon our heads and most people are grotesquely unprepared to cope with it."[3]

As one who teaches in the world of helping professionals, I find myself constantly shocked by statistics that point to the changes going on around us. As you begin to assess change in your life, do not overlook the changes that are happening in your world and may effect your work as human service professionals.

Consider that in 1950 70% of the families in America were headed by a male bread-winner who was the sole support. In 1985 that figure had dropped to 4%.[4]

Fifty-two percent of American women of working age do just that, outside of the home (and then usually come home to their second job . . . taking care of the family and hearth!). This is nine times the figure in 1900. Six out of ten mothers now work opposed to four out of ten just fifteen years ago.[5]

Parents are starting their youngsters in organized play groups, nursery schools, gymnastics, music, and dance classes by the ripe old age of two. Psychologists are now seeing problems with some of these highly structured children as they reach adolescence and doctors report four year olds with peptic ulcers.[6]

The problems and challenges of our aging population are widely talked about. In the next quarter century, the fastest growing age group will be those over 85. By 2030, one in five Americans will be over 65. By 2050 we will have one million people 100 years or older!.[7]

As substance abuse grows, we are beginning to accumulate statistics on the children of one such category, the 28 million offspring of alcoholics. Seven million of these are under age 18. Sons of alcoholics are four times more likely to become alcoholics than other children. Daughters of alcoholic mothers are three times more likely to follow the pattern. Up to 35% of children of alcoholics choose a mate with the same problem. Abnormally high numbers of children of alcoholics go through the juvenile justice systems and mental health facilities. Alcohol is a factor in up to 90% of child abuse cases. Alcoholic's children may be prone to learning disorders, anorexia, frantic over-achievement and suicide.[8]

Not all of us must deal with the ramifications of all these trends and changes, but all of us must deal with some of them.

Helping professionals must be constantly alert to change, having a "Plan B" ready to swing into action to meet emerging needs. Such a need for critical response takes its toll, but as people in the business of caring for others, we tend to minimize the personal toll and focus our energies on the acts necessary to take care of "them."

Such denial of the effect these changes have on us and the drain they are extolling, can cause buried but mounting pressure that can begin to manifest itself in many physical, mental, or emotional symptoms. Take time to reflect on the changes that surround you that have affected your work, its pace, and its pressure. Then take time, possibly with a caring friend, to examine the personal toll it may have had on you. Simply identifying pressure points can be the start of relieving them and moving on to a more health-filled life.

THE CONSTANCY OF CHANGE . . .

In his marvelous book Living, Loving, and Learning,[9] Leo Busgalia quotes from a Hebraic holy book, The Kabala:

> "Man must see that nothing really is but that everything is always becoming and changing. Nothing stands still. Everything is being born, growing and dying. The very instant a thing reaches its height, it begins to decline. The law of rhythm is in constant operation. There is no reality. There is no enduring quality, fixity or substantiality in anything. Nothing is permanent but change. Man must see all things evolving from other things and resolving him to other things, a constant action or reaction, inflow or outflow, building up or tearing down, creation or destruction, birth and growth and death. Nothing is real, and nothing endures but change."

One of the constant demands that helping professionals and care givers must deal with, is the reality of change.

When I was a junior in high school my chemistry class visited the Hiram Walker distillery in Peoria, Illinois. I'm sure the purpose of the field trip was to impress us with the process of fermentation, distillation, etc. but I'm sorry to say I can't recall one portion of that lesson.

What I do recall with vivid clarity is the work of one woman who sat in what I remember to be a vast, noisy, high-ceilinged room on a four-legged stool. In front of her was a conveyor belt which carried capped bottles of liquor at a slow pace from her left to her right.

As each bottle passed in front of her she tapped it once with a metal rod the size of a pencil, producing a distinctive "ping." Occasionally the "ping" had a slightly different sound, and she would respond by slowly removing the unique bottle from the conveyor belt and placing it in a carton beside her.

In the ten minutes or so we were near her she never looked up or acknowledged our presence. She simply tapped each bottle at an exact, slow rynthm, looked mesmerized and only being forced on occasion to break her routine by removing an errant container.

I recall wondering what it would take to get her to indicate that she was indeed human and not a robot. I found out, through asking our guide, that she was checking for improperly sealed bottles (such bottles produced a duller "ping") and that she had been working 40 hours a week for nine years doing this same job! When I bluntly asked our guide how one person could stand such a monotonous job for so long, he shared that the worker said she liked it because "It's always the same. There are no surprises."

Thirty years later I still think of that solitary figure on the high stool, "pinging" away, and I wonder how long she held her job!

I also wonder if I was not seeing a real phenomenon — work that deals with almost no change.

It may be that the horror I felt at ever having to deal with such stagnant work may have cemented a determination to seek work as different as possible from this vice-presidency of "pinging," subsequently leading me to human services with its constant change!

I have known people who have come into our business of serving others, or who have been forced into a personal caregiver role who find great difficulty in dealing with constant change.

When, in the early 1980's, governmental funding was cut for many programs, many groups called and asked me to come train their people in what they often described as "crisis" or "stop gap" fundraising.

They explained that they needed immediate but temporary skills of resource development that would tide them over "till things got back to normal."

When I asked them what "normal" was, they impatiently said that was when all the recent changes were recinded and funding support returned to what it had been pre-change.

I was always tempted to ask if they also believed in the tooth fairy, but held my tongue and tried to share, gently, that any resource development skills I would teach would probably be needed permanently, as it was unlikely they'd ever return to the "normal" they envisioned.

Certainly, we encounter some changes which are temporary, but even after they are reversed, we are not <u>exactly</u> the same as we were before.

For the most part, change for helping professionals and caregivers means a whole new set of rules, reactions, and responses.

To maintain our wholistic health it is important to resist any idea of permanence in any part of our life — home, work, family, community, etc. Terrible anger and anxiety can result from an expectation of things remaining constant and predictable.

I once worked with an older gentleman who went into a tailspin when anything would change. Rearrangement of furniture, sudden crisis that demanded response, schedule changes, or multiple time demands produced a panic reaction of anger, frustration, mental paralysis, and emotional outbursts. He frequently got stuck in "denial" of the need for change and became a source of real trouble because of his inability to adapt and function.

To try to work with the problem, I assigned him volunteer work that was as routine (and to most people, dull) as possible. I also prayed a lot that nothing unusual would happen while he was performing his duties. Since this was primarily mailroom work (stuffing envelopes!) it remained fairly acceptable to him.

A psychologist I spoke with suggested the man's need was for a no-risk, guaranteed success, and his outbursts signaled a personality disorder.

Frequently organizations adopt a variance of this same disorder by refusing to change established patterns. "But we always" and "but we never" statements shoot down any new ideas which propose change. Creative people who try to impact such organizations frequently leave after a few times of being shot down. What is left behind is a stagnating and decaying organization that cannot figure out why its ranks, potency, and influence are declining. (If you are a part of such an organization be aware of the stress that causes you!)

When people block or refuse to acknowledge the constancy of change, they will find themselves expending their energy on fruitless efforts of denial, anger, and the pursuit of the status quo.

Change is a fact of life. It is the process of evolving and becoming and will not be denied. To set yourself up with an expectation that today's changes will finally "flatten out" to produce permanency is to set yourself up for disappointment. Healthy people accept change as it comes, doing the best job they can with new realities and adapting, even if that means contortion! to life as it is.

I'm convinced everyone needs to map out life in pencil, with an eraser ever at the ready!

THE PARADOX OF CHANGE ...

I'd like to quickly point out a paradox that fascinates me in regard to change: EVERY CHANGE BEGINS WITH AN ENDING.

For something to begin anew (change) something else must come to an end. This ending is really a loss of something that was and can be either minor or major.

In the cumulative change section of this chapter, I mentioned the closing of your favorite store as one change you might encounter mixed in with many others. Obviously, this is not what we would list as a major loss, unless, of course, you had owned the store, but it certainly is a change!

To look at it as the change occurs, we see that the store's closing really means an end to the store's existence as you knew it, even when new owners take over at the same site, and therefore a loss of the familiar. If you have been shopping in this store for several years, you knew where everything was, what specialities they offered, the personnel assisting you, even the smells and "feel" of the store itself.

New owners will bring about changes that make you have to hunt for your favorite cereal, possibly do without a valued specialty and adjust to new personnel. The emotions that are triggered by such changes evoke feelings of loss of control over your surroundings and possibly even grief at the loss of relationships you enjoyed with the people who had worked there.

If all this occurs over the relatively minor stressor of a store closing, imagine on a greater scale the feelings of loss that are felt when there is an ending to the life of someone close to you, a dear relationship, a home, a job, etc. Each brings about major changes in your life, and each change is begun by an ending.

To dig even deeper into a closely related paradox, each change signals a start of something new, therefore there is the paradox that states: FOR SOMETHING NEW TO BEGIN, SOMETHING OLD MUST END.

These related paradoxes, if unacknowledged, can cause great feelings of uneasiness, imbalance, and confusion. When we realize their existence, we can begin to cope with their seeming ambiguity and incongruency.

When I began my work as an independent trainer I had to say goodbye to my work leading an international charity. The work in that charity had not been satisfying for two years previous to my departure, and I couldn't wait to get on to my new challenge.

Imagine my surprise when I felt real grief at the change! What I'd overlooked was the reality that to start on my new work I had to grieve over the loss of the old — with its routines, people, and identity now removed from my life. The change brought a sense of loss at the same time that it brought new joy and challenge!

ALLOWING A "NEUTRAL" ZONE . . .

Again I must credit the wisdom of Elaine Yarbrough for first pointing out to me the necessity of allowing a neutral period to exist at the time of change in our lives.

We need to find ways to take a step backward and simply click our mind into neutral gear as we gather perspective, say goodbye to what was, and strengthen ourselves peacefully to handle the confusion and subsequent new beginnings that are demanded by change.

We, in the helping professions, are used to squeezing productivity out of every moment, and may find it difficult to allow ourselves some time simply to "be" rather than to "do." It is critical, however, that we develop the art of going into "neutral," and giving ourselves time to adapt, heal, and most importantly, renew. The neutral zone gives us all these gifts.

While still in the hospital, and during a particularly difficult time, I recalled Elaine's words on the importance of a neutral period when a major change occurs. With her encouragement, I felt comfortable in switching my active brain to "off" and simply flowing with the events around me.

Instead of trying to assess what had happened, figure out how it had come about, ascribe blame, or try to decide about my future, I simply gave myself permission to float in time. I became the spectator to life around me, even refusing to make decisions beyond very basic ones and rejecting getting involved in the needs of others. In short, it became a very self-centered period completely foreign to my nature that normally demands long-range thinking, decision making on he spot, and involvement in the problems and lives of everyone around me.

As a person used to much action and mental gymnastics, this "neutral" zone did not come easily. When someone who called to see how I was doing slipped into sharing some organizational problems and asking my advice, I paused and stated that I really couldn't think about that then and felt at peace about sharing my honest need to not have to "fix" everyone.

I am convinced that by allowing myself this neutral period, I aided in my physical and emotional healing dramatically. Instead of jumping right into the actions required for adjusting, when I was already in a highly weakened state, I gave myself a time to catch my breath, to refill the well of my being, and to gather strength for the adjustments I needed to make to a very major change in my life.

When I originally looked at the subject of a neutral zone, I realized I had an immediate bad image of what that looked like. Tragically, I recalled a friend of mine, who after his wife left him and then divorced him, withdrew from life altogether, refusing to make even the simplest decisions, quitting his job, drinking heavily, and eventually living out of his car as he ran away from life in his unresolved grief and anger at his loss. His message was clear — "rescue me" as he chose to allow all meaning to drain from his existence.

This was not a neutral zone. In my friend's case, it was severe depression, mental illness, and an unproductive period in his life because of the illness.

It was important to distinguish between what was happening to my friend and what Elaine was referring to as a neutral zone. To do so, I realized that I had to distinguish between the words productive and unproductive.

A neutral zone, because of its positive ability to refresh and allow you to get in touch with yourself and your feelings, is very productive even though it may not be marked by "works" and "doing." It is therefore, not the opposite of productivity and positive action.

As I have worked with up to 15,000 helping professionals a year through my training seminars, and therefore heard one story after another of the problems they encounter, I have become convinced that the hardest thing for them to deal with is periods of "non-work" that they immediately label "unproductive."

As I urge these people, for instance, to take time to dream, I encounter great resistance through the excuses they use for not dreaming . . . "I simply don't have time." "You don't understand the demands I have on my desk." "I have to quantitate everything I do to my boss, so I couldn't possibly take time for dreaming!"

In each of these excuses, please note that the speaker is blaming someone or something else for their not having time to dream, to create, to visualize, etc. This gets them off the hook from taking control of their time and life and from having to justify to their own "doer" side any time given over to their need to incubate, reflect, or simply "be." Somehow, as helping professionals we brand any time we spend away from active "doing" as self-centered and therefore "bad", even "evil".

Only when we come to peace with our human need for a period of neutrality that is positively self-centered and therefore gets us in touch with ourselves, giving us much needed refilling of the spirit, will we have a vital tool to our whole health and the strength we need to go on helping others. Buddha may have said it best . . . "Don't just do something, sit there!"

I urge you to examine your life for those opportunities you already have for "neutral zones." I personally find that walking or listening to classical music gives me a chance to wipe my thoughts clear and become "neutral." Since I try to do a bit of both of these things each day, I really already have time set into my schedule for renewal.

When major changes occur, I now try to make additional time to have neutral periods to help me deal with the change. I never try

25

to pre-determine just how much time I will need but instead trust that I will know when I've had the time that is "enough."

I urge you to identify those activities and time slots you already have in your life that can provide this much needed neutral time for yourself and to resolve to make as much additional time for major change adjustments as you may need. See these periods as positive and productive. Avoid labeling the lack of work or "doing" in these periods as "unproductive" and release any guilt feelings about being self-centered.

Take a moment now to identify those times you already have in your life that could become needed "neutral zones" for lessor changes. Then identify opportunities you might create for longer neutral zones needed for more major changes.

NEUTRAL ZONE OPPORTUNITIES YOU HAVE ALREADY

— Going to/from work
— Alone time at home
— Alone time at work
— Walking, jogging, etc.
— Listening to music
— Doing hand-work (crafts, etc.)
— After family has gone off in morning and before you must leave
— During sports activities
— Walking the dog
— Pursuing a hobby (photography, sailing, etc.)
— Other: _____

NEUTRAL ZONE OPPORTUNITIES YOU MIGHT CREATE

— Going off by yourself (resort, motel, etc.)
— Taking a day off from work
— Staying home while the family goes off to an event
— Taking a vacation
— Going to a retreat
— Entering into an activity that does not permit you to think about your concerns
— Giving yourself permission not to have to act in relation to a major chance for a length of time
— Other: _____
  _____

I also urge you to identify those settings and/or activities which lend themselves to peaceful reflection and renewal for you. This will

26

be a highly personalized list as everyone finds peace in different settings. Keep your list handy, and when things begin to overwhelm you, look at it and take action to put yourself in touch with either a setting or activity which can set the stage for your own coping mechanisms.

SETTINGS	ACTIVITIES WHICH REFRESH
Near water	Fishing
Mountains	Golfing (and all sports)
Woods	Reading
The theatre	Walking
Parents' home	Exercising
Golf course	Dancing
Home of a friend	Photography
A museum	Singing
Church	Attending church
Retreat center	Studying the Bible
Campus	Writing
A farm	Sewing
A hotel	Talking with friends
Other: _____	Giving a party
_____	Cooking
	Not cooking (eating out!!)
	Painting (canvas or walls!!)
	Sailing
	Other: _____
	_____

As you look at these lists you will note that your reaction to some is that they sound wonderful, and to others that they sound awful. Remember that a neutral zone does not necessarily mean you are doing nothing at all — simply nothing related to your change other than gathering strength to adapt. This explains why the person who works hard to give a party because that is a real point of renewal can actually be refreshed after the event. They have given themselves permission to let a change in another part of their life remain in the "neutral zone" while they concentrate on something else.

Others of you will find a need to do little or nothing during your neutral zone. Both approaches are "right" if they accomplish the goal of providing renewal and refilling.

LETTING GO ...

One of the major stumbling blocks to change and adjusting to it, seems to be the ability to really "let go."

Very often, helping professionals I deal with regale me with horror stories from their agency or program regarding imposed changes. Funding, administrative demands, personnel changes, etc. have made their job impossible, they share, and they ask me to tell them what to do.

I have noticed, however, that many of these people, when I offer suggestions, immediately reject all possible solutions, branding them as "impossible in my case" and beginning their responses with such poor-me phrases as "But I never," "But I always," or "Yea but ... " At that point, I know that I am dealing with someone who really only wants to prove that nothing can be done, that nothing good can come from their predicament, and that they are justified in their anger, depression, or resistance.

The root of their problem is not the change itself, but their refusal to let go of what was ... what existed before the change.

Before I go on, let me hasten to share that I am not being judgmental about such people, because in the late 1970's I was doing exactly the same thing. I had been with an organization for six years and had been frustrated for the last two as I constantly bumped my head on people above me who, though dedicated and well-meaning, knew very little about personnel or volunteer management.

Much of my time during those last two years was spent simply trying to survive, to somehow have my ideas heard, and to manage my paid and non-paid staff in an enabling rather than disabling way. Although I didn't realize what was happening at the time, almost every "game" in the book was being thrown at me, in the hope, I suppose, that I would become discouraged enough to leave.

As I spent my energies on resisting such a move and trying to provide the best and clearest direction for the innumerable volunteers somehwere under my management umbrella across the nation, I failed to notice the personal toll the effort was taking. In my determination to serve "them" I was doing great disservice to myself.

One symptom of this toll was that I quietly slipped into an Eeyore pattern (The sourpuss donkey in "Winnie the Pooh" stories), rejecting any suggestions of how to make my work environment better. "You just don't understand how bad it is," or "that wouldn't work with ... " were my answers to the suggestions offered by "experts" I cornered for advice.

28

In reality, I was stuck in the grief stage of denial, refusing to let go of the way things had once been and the way I felt they should be. ("Gosh, we're all here to help our clients; surely there should be a way to work everything out!")

In 1978 I attended the Volunteer Management Program at the University of Colorado in Boulder under the direction of Marlene Wilson. One of the faculty members was Mike Murray, an excellent trainer whose expertise lies in problem solving for individuals and organizations. Over coffee one morning, I chewed Mike's ear off about my organizational problems. When he offered solid suggestions I promptly rejected them, until in his gentle wisdom, he placed his hand on my shoulder, looked me straight in the eye and said, "Then know when to get off the merry-go-round; you obviously don't want to be on it!"

Suddenly, with Mike's insight, I saw clearly what I was doing . . . refusing to let go of an organization I had loved and work I saw as my "ministry."

In most cases, the reluctance to let go does not result in so drastic a measure as leaving a position but is instead a stage of grief that does not allow a person to adjust to change because of the pain of loss of "what was."

Stop for a moment and think of the major changes in your work or personal life over the past few months. Seeing the steps from change to adjustment as being four-fold: 1) Change, 2) Neutral Zone, 3) Adapting, 4) Adjustment. Where are you in relation to each event? Are there some changes that seem to have you stuck at stage #1 whereby the change has occurred but you have not been able to move through the adaptation steps (or grief steps)? Are you still stuck on denial or anger with any of the changes?

If you find that you are indeed "stuck," examine the possibility that the necessary emotional action of "letting go" has not yet occurred. Look at ways that might enable this stage to proceed. You may wish to discuss your loss and reluctance to let go of what was with a close friend or professional counselor. You may wish to slip into a short neutral zone to allow acceptance to come to you and to gather the strength to adjust.

I find it helpful, when I am having difficulty letting go of something, to visualize my life without it, examining just how that feels. I try to look for all the positive aspects of this "new way of life" and even experience the good feelings that would result. I also look at the negatives that might come from ths new life, studying their consequences and imagine coping measures for each.

In the case of my difficulties many years ago with an organization that was very important to me, I had to visualize myself letting go of it entirely and working in some other capacity. When I did this, I saw myself sharing with others the things I had learned in managing 30,000 volunteers and raising 17 million dollars. As I drew this image more clearly, my present career of training and consulting with volunteer management and resource development professionals began to emerge. In short, I was able to see myself letting go of one phase of my life and moving on to another.

As I examine my life of the past few years, understanding that my hectic travel pace must be a thing of the past for health reasons, I am again faced with letting go of the old image as a constanly on-the-go trainer, yelling "Have flip chart, will travel" in airports! Though my visualizations are not yet totally clear (I'm still allowing myself some neutral time, thank you) I am beginning to see myself moving from helping people to "do" things better, to helping people simply "be" better . . . through more writing and publications, counseling, consulting, and some selected training.

Letting go is not easy. It involves deep examination and introspection of self-image, private perceptions, and distinctions between worth and works. It frequently involves the grief process whose stages are often painful to experience. The pain, however, is a sign of growth, as we move from what was, to new beginnings; from loss to exciting gains.

I read somewhere that people who come to the circus to see the flying trapeze acts do so not to see the artists do the tricks on their swinging bars, but for that split second when everyone holds their breath as the artist lets go of one bar so that they can reach for another. The suspense comes while they are suspended in space between the two.

For everyone who encounters major changes in their life, there is a split second, when through sheer determination and accepting risk, we must let go of what we held on to in the past and reach for what is ahead of us in the future, enduring that time period between when we feel we have nothing to hold on to except our faith that the future is ours if we only reach for it.

ROLE CHANGES . . .

"The only thing that remains constant, is change," someone once said, and it is certainly true in the various roles that make up our lives. Three different role change areas repeatedly are pointed to as major sources of stress and concern, and each needs to be examined as a possible trouble spot for us. Again, had I been watching my own life I would have seen that two of the three were occurring in my life simultaneously.

The first comes in the area of our changing roles with both children and parents. It is not uncommon, that at approximately the same time, there are major role changes with the generation above and below a person. At about the time that the last child is leaving the nest, elderly parents move to a point of needing assistance in their lives.

The change of the senior parents from independence to greater dependence causes many adjustments in the minds of those who have, all their lives, looked at their parents as the bedrocks of security and strength. At the same time, children are leaving the nest, pulling away from dependence on their parents and asserting their own independence. This near-paradox causes people caught in the middle to have to shift emotional and often physical gears, hopefully, without offending either generation.

It is often a time of great pain for those "caught in the middle" . . . new definitions for relationships must be hammered out. Periods of uncertainty and anxiety on everyone's part must be adjusted to, and expectations take on new directions as everyone tries to settle into new roles.

As people used to helping others, our first instinct with both generations is to "help," and to try to make the transitions as painless as possible. Unfortunately this may be resented by our children and considered "meddling." In helping our parents we must walk the fine line of helping enough without infringing upon their dignity and the independence they still retain.

A second area of concern is for those role changes which occur at work.

A promotion can cause real stress as we adjust to a new position in relation to the people around us and the work itself. We need to keep in mind that stress comes not just from negative life occurrances, but from positive successes also. A person with a torrent of "good" changes in their lives . . . successes, promotions, additional income, acclaim, etc. . . . can feel as much stress as the person with an accumulation of negative stressors. With that point in mind you may wish to look again at your life changes list to reassess stress.

We gather much support and comfort from our peers, but when a job change creates a new peer group and leaves the other behind, the change can bring tension and confusion. Feelings of not belonging anywhere can, for a time, plague us. Resentment can come unexpectedly from people once considered good friends and supporters. Supervisors can seem strongly threatened as we come a step closer to their position or "territory."

All of these emotional factors can be a part of the larger change of a new role and add additional pressure beyond just trying to adjust to a new job.

A third, obvious role change occurs when a person loses a mate or close companion. Suddenly everything that was shared must now be carried by the remaining partner. This can feel like real abandonment and overwhelmingly demanding. Thoughts of "I can't do all this" and "I can't go on" are common, and a period of grief and adjustment must be endured.

This loss, which ranks at the top of every stress and crisis scale as the most devastating, can come from loss through death, divorce, physical separation (military duty, etc.), job transfer, etc.

When such a heavy change occurs, we must first recognize its impact on all aspects of our lives and work through the changes it has created.

Role changes and reversals occur at different stages of our lives. We can come to peace with them more quickly by recognizing their impact and understanding them as a natural part of the transitions of life. Rather than focusing on what was, we need to move on to what now is the new reality and develop coping mechanisms to handle them.

ATTITUDES TOWARD CHANGE ...

Recently, as my father's health began to fail beyond my mother's ability to provide all his care, they were put in touch with a social worker to help them arrange home health care. Fortunately for them, the social worker was creative, positive, and resourceful and found ways to work with, and sometimes around, the system to provide the help needed.

Once, during an initial interview, the worker confided her frustration and real anger at the programatic cuts that had so reduced the assistance available to the elderly. Obviously this "people helper" had recognized the changes in support for her clients and had come up with creative ways to find needed help for those she cared for so deeply.

Her attitude was positive and upbeat; therefore, her energies were being directed to solving problems rather than blaming.

In a parallel incident with a close friend trying to arrange home care for her elderly mother, the social worker and health professionals she spoke with had found a different way to deal with the same frustrations. Their answer to anything my friend asked about Meals on Wheels, home nursing, home aides, etc. was an emphatic, "It just can't be done!"

Tragically, there are many people in our helping professions who, out of sheer frustration at budget cuts, beaurocracy, red tape, and puny administrative attitudes have simply shut themselves down, drawing a cloke of negativism around them in an attempt to avoid one more failure at providing client needs.

My guess is that the people my friend encountered had not recognized the personal toll changes in their work environment had brought them. Their coping response was to play Eeyore, the doomsaying donkey of "Winnie the Pooh" fame, and deny that anything positive could happen. In a way, they were playing a variation of the blame game, washing their hands of responsibility for helping clients by insisting and even aiding in the process of impossibility, while blaming all failures on the "others" who had caused the circumstances.

In these two cases, the actual circumstances of programs, cuts, frustrations, etc. were the same . . . both social workers faced the same options for acquiring needed home health care for elderly patients. The only difference was the chosen attitude of each worker . . . one positive, thus seeing the changes as challenges for new solutions, and one negative, seeing the changes as a place to hide from their responsibilities and place blame for failure on "others."

As we seek to survive in the midst of innumerable changes, both in the workplace and in our personal lives, we must not only be cognizant of the effect those changes have on us, but also the attitudes we develop in response to the changes.

Those who choose to foster a positive attitude no matter what the change will have a better chance at accomplishing whatever goals they set AND take a giant step toward a healthfilled, productive life!

CONCLUSION

Changes will always be a part of our lives.

The critical factor is how we react to changes in all aspects of our lives and our realistic appraisal of how these changes effect us.

As I said at the start of this chapter, the greatest change I ever encountered was my colostomy, and I had to look carefully at how it effected all of my dimensions so that I could adapt and cope with the changes it brought about.

In having to assess and adapt to it however, I learned a very valuable lesson I believe will help me to a healthier future. The lesson comes in the form of a new sensitivity to the existance and impact of change on my life.

As I go through life now, I am constantly aware of changes; I assess their impact and examine options for my reactions in order to find the best ways to cope.

I have carefully examined changes in my past to insure that I have not buried any unresolved grief or anger. I look at changes that surround me in my daily and professional lives. I am on the alert for changes in my personal life that effect me and in each case I examine their multilayered impact on my being.

It is as if I am constantly taking my "charge temperature" to insure that I am aware of what's really happening within myself and am able to see any danger signals.

Occassionally I need the help of someone else's perspective when I cannot quite unravel my feelings in response to a particular occurrence. My support system is particularly helpful to me at such times and in each case have been able to help me "sort out" what's going on internally.

As helping professionals we encounter more than our share of challenges to adjust to changes. It is critical that we clearly assess them in all facets of our lives so that we can be equipped with the information we need to cope positively with their effect.

THE SOCIAL READJUSTMENT RATING SCALE

LIFE EVENT	MEAN VALUE
1. Death of spouse	100
2. Divorce	73
3. Marital separation from mate	65
4. Detention in jail or other institution	63
5. Death of a close family member	63
6. Major personal injury or illness	53
7. Marriage	50
8. Being fired at work	47
9. Marital reconciliation with mate	45
10. Retirement from work	45
11. Major change in the health or behavior of a family member	44
12. Pregnancy	40
13. Sexual difficulties	39
14. Gaining a new family member (e.g., through birth, adoption, oldster moving in, etc.)	39
15. Major business readjustment (e.g., merger, reorganization, bankruptcy, etc.)	39
16. Major change in financial state (e.g., a lot worse off or a lot better off than usual)	38
17. Death of a close friend	37
18. Changing to a different line of work	36
19. Major change in the number of arguments with spouse (e.g., either a lot more or a lot less than usual regarding child-rearing, personal habits, etc.)	35
20. Taking on a mortgage greater than $10,000 (e.g., purchasing a home, business, etc.)	31
21. Foreclosure on a mortgage or loan	30
22. Major change in responsibilities at work (e.g., promotion, demotion, lateral transfer)	29
23. Son or daughter leaving home (e.g., marriage, attending college, etc.)	29
24. In-law troubles	29
25. Outstanding personal achievement	28
26. Wife beginning or ceasing work outside the home	26
27. Beginning or ceasing formal schooling	26
28. Major change in living conditions (e.g., building a new home, remodeling, deterioration of home or neighborhood	25
29. Revision of personal habits (dress, manners, associations, etc.)	24
30. Troubles with the boss	23
31. Major change in working hours or conditions	20
32. Change in residence	20
33. Changing to a new school	20
34. Major change in usual type and/or amount of recreation	19
35. Major change in church activities (e.g., a lot more or a lot less than usual)	19
36. Major change in social activities (e.g., clubs, dancing, movies, visiting, etc.)	18
37. Taking on a mortgage or loan less than $10,000 (e.g., purchasing a car, TV, freezer, etc.)	17
38. Major change in sleeping habits (a lot more or a lot less sleep, or change in part of day when asleep)	16
39. Major change in number of family get-togethers (e.g., a lot more or a lot less than usual)	15
40. Major change in eating habits (a lot more or a lot less food intake, or very different meal hours or surroundings)	15
41. Vacation	13
42. Christmas	12
43. Minor violations of the law (e.g., traffic tickets, jaywalking, disturbing the peace, etc.)	11

* Holmes and Rahe Social Readjustment Rating Scale.
  Journal of Psychosomatic Research, 1967

There seems to be a definite relationship between life change and physical illness. Holmes and Rahe interpret total scores:

Score for previous year:	Illness probability in next 2 years:
Less than 150 (low stress)	Low
150-199 (mild stress)	30%
200-299 (moderate stress)	50%
300 or more (major stress)	80%

LIFE EVENTS CHECKLIST DURING LAST YEAR
Rate each as positive, negative, or neutral.

FAMILY	+	−	WHEN OCCURRED? (MONTH)
Death of a spouse			
Divorce			
Marital separation			
Death of a child			
Death of a close family member			
Marriage			
Engagement			
Health change of family member			
Child moves out			
Youngest child off to college			
In-law trouble			
Job change of spouse			
Change in number of family gatherings			
Parent illness or dependence			
Estrangement with family member			
Close family member substance abuse			
Change in number of arguments with spouse			
Separation from spouse due to travel/work			
Marriage of a child			
Family member comes to live with you			
New child in family			
Other:			

PERSONAL LIFE	+	−	WHEN OCCURRED? (MONTH)
Personal injury or illness			
Death of a close friend			
Estrangement from close friend			
Close friend moves away			
Move to new location			
Change in time to be alone			
Change in personal habits			
Change of schools			
Change in recreation			
Change in religious activities			
Change in social activities			
Change in sleeping habits			
Change in exercise habits			
Change in eating habits			
Weight gain or loss			
Leaving home for the first time			
Loss of pet			
Birthday			
Change in time with friends			
New goals set			
New insight into self			
Change in amount of time for "play"			
Other:			

SEXUAL   +   –   WHEN OCCURRED? (MONTH)

Pregnancy
Sex difficulties
Confusion over sexual orientation/preference
Abortion
New sexual experiences
Other:

FINANCIAL   +   –   WHEN OCCURRED? (MONTH)

Forclosure of loan or mortgage
Take on indebtedness
Pay off indebtedness
Change in income
Sudden wealth or money gift
Sudden money crunch
Financial uncertainty
Investment loss
Difficulty with IRS
Other:

LEGAL   +   –   WHEN OCCURRED? (MONTH)

Jail term
Trial
Minor violation with law
Being sued
Sueing others
Other:

JOB RELATED	+	−	WHEN OCCURRED? (MONTH)
Fired			
Changed jobs			
Promoted			
Increased responsibility			
Budget cut			
Programatic changes			
Retirement			
New line of work			
Trouble with boss			
Trouble with peers			
Trouble with subordinates			
Change work hours or conditions			
Change of work site			
Vacation			
Overtime			
Client/patient numbers increase			
Client/patient numbers decrease			
Difficulty with volunteer			
Volunteer/staff problems			
Set goals and objectives			
Work timelines too short			
Unclear job description			
Lack of peers close by			
Recognition from administration			
Lack of recognition for work			
Negative feedback on job review			
Poor communication between work levels			
No real direction from above			
Unclear mission of agency/organization			
Constant crisis management			
Job uncertain (political, appointment, etc.)			
Once satisfying work now tedious			
Unreasonable demands			
Major project completed			
Major project begun			
Reduced support staff			
New supervisor			
Other:			

39

CHAPTER I
END NOTES

1. Holmes, Thomas and Rahe, Richard. *Social Readjustment Scale,* Journal of Psychosomatic Research, 1967.

2. Vineyard, Sue. *Finding Your Way Through The Maze of Volunteer Management,* Heritage Arts. Downers Grove, IL. 1981.

3. Bridges, William. *Transitions.* Addison Wesley Pub., Reading, MA. 1980.

4. Today's Education. NEA. 1986-87.

5. Ibid.

6. Ibid.

7. Ibid.

8. Ibid.

9. Buscaglia, Leo. *Living, Loving, and Learning.* Fawcett Columbine, NY. 1982.

CHAPTER II

THE QUIET KILLERS

GRIEF . . .

One of the greatest insights that I am still exploring, and experiencing, is the phenomenon known to us all . . . that of grief.

At a younger age, when grief was spoken of, I thought immediately of the death of someone, counting myself lucky that I had not experienced it in my close family or among dear friends. Then, when I was in Junior High School a girl I had met through church affiliations died of leukemia, and I attended my first funeral and experienced my first identifiable grief.

Through my sadness at the loss of my friend I was also startled to note that the feelings I was experiencing were not unfamiliar to me at all. They mirrored the various feelings I had experienced as my father was trasferred frequently in his sales positions, and I had had to uproot from home, school, and friends. It was at this time, therefore, that I realzed that grief comes not just through death, but more simply, the loss of anything meaningful to you.

In looking back at what compounded my health problems, far

beyond physical weaknesses that were inherited, I realize that grief ... most of it unresolved ... was a great contributing factor.

Throughout my life, as I had experienced numerous endings of relationships and experiences which were very important to me, I simply gritted my teeth and rushed headlong on paying little attention to the feelings of loss. In doing so I was storing up a pile of unresolved grief experiences that were slowly erroding my health and well being.

I had not really ever come to peace with the loss of my daughter-in-law, a close friend of over 20 years, my one son's handicap, my leaving an organization that I dearly loved, the loss of relationships in that organization, the assurance of my parent's or husband's health.

As each had occurred in my life, my way of handling them was to put on a happy face, bury myself in my travel schedule, and keep a stiff upper lip. I had never given myself time to have a neutral zone in which to examine my feelings and express them openly. Even experiences I had had in my work with the national charity which caused me to deal occasionally with dying children, had not truly been resolved. I rejected the sadness I might feel in thinking of any of these occurances, so I simply did not think about them!

I am trying to experience grief differently these days, as I know it is far more healthy for me to do so. I still find it a struggle, but I know that I am not alone as I have heard from so many people who have written to share the grief and adjustments they are going through.

I write and edit a newsletter (cleverly titled "Grapevine" with my last name!) which is an informal, bi-monthly creation going to people in the field of human services and volunteer administration. It shares whatever people have sent in regarding our work plus concerns, tidbits, humor, personal information and anything else I feel is of interest to the readership across the US and Canada. Through this medium I have briefly shared wih people my health experiences.

Amidst the pile of well-wishes from Grapeviners, certain notes stand out ... those from people with similar or even identical incidents who write to say "You're not alone!" I have noticed a theme among the letters, that of the writers being in various stages of grief. A friend wrote about her mastectomy and her determination to hold tight to those brief moments of hope when the clouds in her life part and a ray of sunshine pops in. Another wrote to share her successes since having a colostomy, but she ended her letter with "I still struggle, however, with depression and panic at my situation and work daily on adjusting to the loss of normalcy." A third wrote to share his anger at what had happened to him (a colostomy) and the reaction of people around him who felt, since it has been a reality or five years, that he should be totally adjusted to it by now.

Each of these people is experiencing one of the stages of grief and none of them are referring to loss of life, but loss of what was and is no longer.

As caregivers, we experience in our work life, many forms of losses . . . from patient and client losses to death, despair, disintegration, etc.; from loss of the tools (money, procedures, permissions, etc.) to carry out the best possible work, and from losses of wonderful co-workers who leave under good conditions, or sadly, under those of burnout, disenchantment or detachment.

When we add losses in our personal and social lives, we compound those pressures and tensions that build in us, possibly pushing us closer to the brink of breakdown, burnout, or physical illness.

The only way I know of to lessen this grip of grief on ourselves is to first understand the process of grief. There is a normal, good grief process that needs to be experienced at times of loss, and we need to assess our own lives in relation to that process.

In his wonderful little book called Good Grief,[1] Pastor Granger Westburg shares his list of ten natural stages of grief. He cautions, wisely, that not everyone will experience the ten in his listed order, but the various stages usually occur as people work their way from darkness to light.

His ten stages are:

1. *State of Shock:* Numbness, temporarily anesthetized; keeps us from having to face grim reality all at once.
2. *Expressing Emotion:* When we realize how dreadful the event is, our emotions pour forth. Many people deny themselves this stage, trying to keep their emotions inside. Such a tactic is disastrous!
3. *Depression and loneliness:* A feeling of total isolation and abandonment. We are sure no one has ever felt this awful before and no one understands our grief. A rejection of God is not uncommon here as a feeling of "If there is a God He would have prevented this from happening" overtakes the person.
4. *Physical Symptoms:* (Pastor Westburg conducted a survey at a hospital he was working with to identify how many patients had experienced a grief situation during the year previous to their admittance . . . he was startled to find that ⅔ of the

43

patients had just such an occurrence in their history!) Immediately following a major loss, sleeplessness, digestive tract problems, headaches, muscle spasms, etc. are common complaints.

5. *Panic:* Difficulty concentrating; paralyzed with fear, etc.
6. *Anger and Resentment:* Wanting someone to blame; lashing out; even anger at the time of death at the person who has died and abandoned them.
7. *Resisting Returning:* Feelings of being disloyal if their life returns to normal, mundane things. Rejection of happiness as somehow not befitting the circumstance.
8. *Guilt:* Feeling there was more that we could have done for the person or situation; feeling we did "wrong" things that brought problems about, etc.
9. *Gradually Hope Comes Through:* Those at first infrequent times, when, in the midst of despair, a little ray of hope shines through; a lightening of the burden and the tension occurs.
10. *We Struggle to Affirm Reality:* Wisely Westburg does not call this final stage the "return to normal," for with any loss, life is never exactly the same was it was before. Instead this phase signals a reentry into living each day, no longer consumed with thoughts of the loss, but functioning in a healthy, aware manner, possibly sadder but wiser . . . and certainly hopeful once again.

As I read through the author's stages, I recognize that I am still working through my own grief at the loss of Sue Vineyard as she once was . . . running from town to town, interacting and training with thousands of people annually, gathering equal acclaim and exhaustion along the road. Because I so closely identified myself with the work I did, it has been hard to say no to so many fine clients who want me to squeeze in "just a day or two" in my schedule for the next few years.

The easy part was determining I would only do a few training sessions each year (down from 50-60); the hard part is carrying forth on this determination when a friend or a particularly needy client calls and works hard to get me to change my "no" to a "yes." I go through feelings of guilt after hearing their pleadings, and the grief can engulf me all over again when I hang up the phone.

I recognize that I am grieving at several levels simultaneously: grief at the loss of ability to continue doing what I do best (training) in the same amount as before; grief at the loss of opportunities I will have to interact with dear friends across the country or to acquire many new ones; and finally, but not unimportantly the loss of financial security for my family (when I don't train folks, I don't get paid!).

In confronting these levels, I at first denied the necessity for the change of my work patterns ("When I get back to my normal routine, all will be well . . . "). I moved from that to anger that this had happened . . . anger directed at times at others, at times at myself. Next came depression and loneliness, then panic and guilt, then emotion and new physical symptoms, fear of returning, and finally sprinkles of hope and reentry into life as it now must be.

In this final stage I was able to make new plans for the future and enjoy each day given me, even when flashbacks and feelings of sadness at having to say no came over me.

Grief is a part of all of our lives. As caregivers I believe we experience more grief that the average person through our work in trying to serve others. Human services is an inexact science at best, with many disappointments, setbacks and losses built into it. When we are also faced with losses in our personal lives, the tension mounts and can exact a high toll if not dealt with in a healthy way.

I urge all of you to look carefully at losses in your life, assessing your own grief stage with each and working to bring them to a hope-filled commitment to life, to love, and to faith.

BURNOUT . . .

I worked up to a major burnout in the late seventies, by experiencing several "small burns," if there are such things.

After serving as an officer in a local service organization, on the board of a community Youth Center and being Superintendent of a church school simultaneously, I experienced exhaustion after a major project, becoming physically ill and mentally fatigued. The problem was a familiar one, especially to young mothers with active children at home . . . too many tasks and demands in too short a time span.

At the time I thought . . . "Ah, so this is what burnout is . . . and after a few days rest, I returned to the same old pace, propping myself up with a little better spacing of activities, which seemed to "cure" what ailed me.

Actually what I was experiencing was a taste of burnout, but nothing like the real thing, which I found out painfully in the late 1970's.

I have mentioned several incidents elsewhere in this work about my time with a charity for which I was National Director and to which I was totally devoted. I mention this last factor because I feel it has a lot to do with the severity of burnout, as those of us who bring total commitment to our work are more likely to ignore the first signs of burnout in our zeal to "hang in there" and save the world through our cause.

Let me first paint a picture of the demands I was experiencing, which, I suspect are similar (sometimes much less than) those many of you are feeling at the present time.

I had risen very quickly through the ranks of local, state, midwest and finally national directorships of the charity. No training or job description was provided for any of the levels . . . it was very much a matter of "you'll figure it out!" I stopped the list of 52 staff members scattered around the country with just two people above me . . . the head of the resources department and the Executive Director.

During my tenure 30,000 volunteers worked to mobilize up to 100,000 participants in a major fundraising event supported by one million sponsors each year. This in turn translated into helping one million clients, mostly impoverished children worldwide, annually.

The event we focused on had peaked in my third year (of six) and was on a downward swing. My plea for more diversified fundraising was going unheeded and met with an attitude of "just work harder and it will generate more money." I was also in charge of training and materials development. I worked in Chicago, the headquarters was in California, and all my people were spread out across the nation, giving us about three face to face meetings per year.

My boss was an amazing public speaker and individual fund raiser, motivating others to action. He was by his own admission (much later), someone completely mystified by principles of management. It took me almost two years to convince him and a second supervisor who once was my immediate boss, to record their knowledge of the charity in general and our fundraiser specifically in writing (they carried it in their heads!). I finally simply wrote the first operations manual on my own time and handed it in. Both of my bosses were amazed at its length and finally admitted it was probably needed. I was also told this action was "out of line."

In hindsight I realize that I became the focus of masterful game playing as I became more strident in demands for training, information sharing, diversification, allowing the ranks to create and make decisions, long range planning, job designs, simpified management structure (at one time there were 11 levels of jobs among 40 people!) and involvement in decisions by the people to be effected. In short, I was crying for appropriate management functioning of planning, organizing, staffing, supervising, and evaluating.

The louder I cried, the more I was told I was "not a good team player," that I was a negative influence on the staff, 90% of which were volunteers; that I simply didn't have all the facts and therefore couldn't be in a position to make judgments. When I seemed to be close to winning a discussion, the focus was shifted to me personally and off the subject at hand.

When I asked for the time and money to attend the first level Volunteer Management Workshop at the University of Colorado[2] in 1978 to acquire more skills, I was first told there was no money in the budget for it. I thought about it for a while then decided to pay for it out of my own pocket. When I shared this I was told I could not have the time off. I then decided to take my vacation time to attend. I was then told the training was imappropriate, and I simply could not attend.

I went anyway, learned greatly and confirmed my own instincts more in that week than ever before. It was at that conference that I discussed my frustrations with Marlene Wilson and Mike Murray, and they caused me to consider leaving the charity as an option.

When I requested permission to attend Level II the following February my boss insisted that he attend with me. A pattern developed . . . whenever Marlene was leading a training session, my boss called me out of the room to discuss business; when anyone else led a workshop, he constantly side-commented to me either how poor the trainer was or how inappropriate the content.

The final straw came when he asked that I meet him in his room to discuss a recent meeting I had tried to have with my people from around the country. He had asked to attend that meeting and take 30 minutes of my tight agenda time. After he actually took 3½ hours on budget(!) my people were furious, and let him know this later. As I tried to get him to see that their anger was directed at the misuse of time, he interrupted with a personal comment that I reminded him of his mother who was unkind to his father and went on to make bizarre remarks about my relationship to my husband.

I can recall getting up from that meeting and taking the elevator to the first floor of the conference center. When the doors opened, Marlene Wilson was standing there, and I can recall the look of horror on her face as she looked at me. She took me gently to the side, asking what had just happened. When I tried to explain, she sat me down and implored me to look carefully at the toll it was taking on me to stay in my position.

What I did not realize was what she saw was a sheet-white, trembling, glazed-eyed person barely able to recognize her surroundings. I had totally burned out.

Beyond what Marlene could see I was experiencing classic symptoms . . . nausea, muscle spasms, fatigue, difficulty in concentrating, colon spasms, diarrhea, nervousness, sleeplessness and impatience.

I had hung on for over two years convinced that the cause of dying children was so compelling that I had to find a way to work around the incompetence of the management above me. I had focused on the commitment of my immediate boss and his own devotion to our clients, missing the point that meaning well is not enough. I ignored all the warning signals my body was giving out and instead focused on my own "should list" regarding my work.

I felt drained, unappreciated, exhausted, frustrated, and on overload. I'd worked for 11 straight weeks without a day off and still I could not keep up with demands. The more appreciation and acclaim I got from below me the less I got from above. I felt like a human guinea pig on one of those exercise wheels, running faster and faster but getting nowhere.

The only bright spot in all this was the timing of my final encounter with my boss ... at level II at the University of Colorado where Marlene Wilson picked up the pieces as I emerged from the elevator and begged me to see what my job was doing to me. I can recall her impassioned plea to me to "get out of that job before it kills you or at the very least drives you from the field ... we can't afford to lose you!"

Though still in shock, I wrote my letter of resignation on the plane going home the next day. I'd like to tell you that that brought an immediate flood of relief, but actually I was so burned out it accentuated a feeling of insecurity (was I doing the right thing?), and self-doubt (maybe I'm the one who is wrong, crazy ... and where do I go from here? Who nees a burned out, probaly talent-less mother in her 40's anyway?!?).

My story might have a slightly different scenario from other readers, but as I have traveled around the world listening to burnout stories of hundreds of others in the helping professions, commonalities jump out at me.

About a year ago I began asking my audiences who among them had experienced or were now experiencing symptoms of burnout, and was horrified to see over 80% of the hands go up! This is a deplorable rate and a terrible statement about our professions, so geared to helping others.

To me it says very loudly, that we must begin to concentrate on helping ourselves and one another become more aware of what is going on inside of us and to find ways to safeguard our wholistic health so that we can prevent or reduce harmful symptoms that could either diminish our effectiveness or rob us of our very life.

In helping professions, we have, by necessity, concentrated on how to "do" things better ... now we must concentrate on how to "be" better, thereby insuring our longer impact on the lives of others and a healthier relationship with ourselves.

BURNOUT SYMPTOMS

As I look back at my own burnout experience, I was demonstrating some of the classic burnout symptoms described by Christina Maslach in her book Burnout . . . The Cost of Caring[3]

1. *Emotional Exhaustion* — feeling drained and used up; unable to give of self to others. Desire to reduce contact with people to bare minimum to get job done.
2. *Depersonalization* — anticipating worst from others; feeling contemptuous toward those who "intrude" with demands; caring less about work results. Negativism.
3. *Reduced Personal Accomplishment* — being down on oneself; doubting own worth and work; feeling guilty about feelings toward others; gnawing sense of inadequacy. Depression.

Obviously, a person does not have to feel all of the symptoms described above to be in or close to burnout. A majority of them, however, should signal a warning so that you can take steps to reduce the problem.

Are you at risk for burnout? Does your work situation cause you to:

1. Deal with many people over extended periods of time?
2. Always be concerned, warm, and caring?
3. Become too involved in clients or workers woes and to sometimes feel overwhelmed by them?
4. Feel a lack of rapport and support among your co-workers?
5. Have an excess of paperwork?
6. Have the frustration of red tape?
7. Focus on people rather than situations?
8. See people only when there are problems?
9. Have little feedback?
10. Provide "instant cures"?
11. Follow illogical rules or procedures?
12. Deal with problems once your own? (alcoholism, loss of child, etc.)
13. Work in an undesirable setting?
14. Be overloaded with assignments?
15. Constantly have to juggle priorities?
16. Have little control over decisions/results that effect you?
17. Deal with unclear goals?

If you recognize characteristics of your job in a number of these, BEWARE of an escalating overload — too much being asked of you and too little returned. The frequency of the situations give a clearer picture of burnout potential. There is a high burnout probability if such things are chronic as chronic problems take a much higher toll on a person.

Had I examined my situation in the late 70s carefully, I would have seen the pressure points before they became overwhelming. I know now that there is a tool by which to measure burnout (Maslach's Burnout Inventory,[4] created with Susan Jackson) that could have predicted my eventual circumstance, and taking it would have helped me make an appropriate decision much earlier than I did.

I am certain that my effectiveness during the last two years of my tenure with the charity were reduced in direct proportion to the energy I was having to direct toward simply surviving. To prevent burnout in the future, I constantly check with myself and others for symptoms. I listen to my body signals for signs that I might be in trouble and am much more aware of the stressors that can lead to burnout.

To help readers also be aware of these little warning flags, let me share some of the learnings we can glean from those who have written on the subject of burnout.

Maslach tells us that when caregivers begin to burnout they tend to blame people for the problems (either the provider — often themselves — or the recipient of the care) for spoiling the ideal relationship between giver and recipient.

We need to focus on what is really causing the problem, to look at the situation and to analyze it carefully. In my case an analysis would have revealed an ineffective management that could do nothing but thwart work. Uunclear mission, non-existant or garbled job designs, gamesplaying, etc. were the norms for the organization . . . an impossible situation.

We need to look at what tasks are expected to be done and why. What setting is the work to be done in? What limitations and constraints exist due to rules? What norms exist, what expectations, etc.?

One Achilles' heel that caregivers seem to have is their tendency to personalize the whole world — to see things as people rather than situations. This frequently leads to blaming ourselves for failures. Instead of seeing that a reporting system in an agency is cumbersome, frequently caregivers focus on the person who must impose the system, seeing them as a personal adversary out to get them.

Burnout is usually a response to chronic rather than occasional stress, so there is a pile-on factor which is common in many of our programs and work situations. Unfortunately, caregivers tend to think they are the only ones with this problem so they try to hide it behind bravado and pretend happiness when they truly feel like a weak link or a complainer. Add to this the fact that most caregivers work in an institutional setting which tends to blame people not systems, and you can see the makings of many potential burnout senarios!

What a person brings to their work situation is just as critical as what the work brings to them. In looking at the burnout question, we must factor in personal motivations, needs, values, self-esteem, emotional expressiveness and control, plus personal style.

I was interested in some research that Maslach and Jackson [5] did to establish patterns of burnout personalities amongst caregivers . . .

Sex: Men and women are about equal but with different characteristics: Women are more likely to have emotional exhaustion more intensely while men are more likely to have depersonalization and callous feelings about people they work with.

Ethnic Background: Blacks seem to experience burnout less than whites.

Age: Younger workers tend to burnout faster than older ones.

Marital and Family Status: Singles experience more burnout than married people. Divorced providers fall in the middle between burnout rates of single or married people. Burnout seems to be less for professional helpers with children.

Education: This varies with the job though a pattern of higher education- higher expectations exists.

THE EFFECTS OF BURNOUT . . .

It is helpful to understand the various effects burnout can have on us wholistically. A partial list includes:

1. *Physical exhaustion* . . . wound up tensely, unable to relax or sleep; bad dreams or nightmares; unnamed fears that something will go wrong. Illness may follow . . . lingering colds, "sinus" problems or headaches, ulcers, neck and back problems, digestive problems, etc. are frequent complaints.

2. *Psychological exhaustion* . . . lack of self-esteem, guilt, "shoulds and oughts'" depression; easily irritated and angry. Hero-martyr Syndrome ("I'm the only one who can do it").

3. *Job Performance* . . . less effective, creative, productive. Poor judgments. Co-workers often demoralized in domino effect.

4. *Family* . . . irritable and impatient at home. Increased bickering, less able to give to other family members, to listen to problems. Desire for solitude rather than bonding. Often feel greater demands for attention (in competition with their work) from family members feeling neglected. May set up unrealistic standards for family members (ie: Ministers with perfect kids; teachers with A student children, etc.). Schedules may be disrupted at any time by on-call status . . . never fully relaxed at home therefore.

STRESS . . .

In thinking over the burnout experience that placed so many physical and emotional demands on me, I realize that it differs subtly from my latest bout that came from a broader spectrum known by most lay people as "stress."

The burnout I experienced was focused totally on problems in the work site, while my latest impacted me from all sides . . . work, relationships, personal crisis, and accumulated stressors.

In the first part of this book I chronicled the eventual outcome, a ruptured colon, a colostomy, and severe, life-threatening peritinitis. A litany of pressure points were pressing on me for many years . . . job stress as it related to constant traveling, performing, being evaluated every time I worked, an overactive calendar and an inability to say no to those who wanted "just five minutes" of my time.

Pressure also came from disappointments in close personal relationships not living up to my ill-founded preconceptions.

Health crises among those I loved came in the form of cancer, Parkinson's disease, strokes, and a heart attack and persisted as chronic concerns.

A piling on effect dumped its stress on me when, in a one week period my husband suffered a heart attack, my younger son was in a bad accident, and our family room flooded! Within six weeks of this time period, I added one wedding, one son's separation, cancer surgery for my father, and a stroke for my mother — plus large financial debt.

Is it any wonder that weekly I was fighting spastic bowel syndrome, diverticulitis, difficulty sleeping, muscle spasms, ulcers, and almost constant pain from one or more of these symptoms? Not really.

Through it all, I continued on with my work, training and entertaining audiences in a manner that brought on the added positive stress (called eustress) of acclaim and statements of "Boy you really have it all together!" Tragically, this perception of me by others added to the pressure, because it gave me the feeling of false security and a desire to live up to their appraisal of me.

In looking back at this script, the events on a hot July 5th in the emergency room of my local hospital should have come as no surprise. The only surprise might be that it took so many years before it all came crashing down on me!

Since that fateful July day, I have done a great deal of reading on stress to try to truly understand all its facets and to internalize that learning as never before in order to use it to prevent reoccurrances.

How Our Body Responds . . .

Our body is primed to respond to stressors . . . those events that impact us physically. In days of old the proper response to a threat was to grab a spear and fight off the invader.

Unfortunately, no reprograming of the body was possible even after our stressors changed. It is relatively rare for us to be attacked by tigers, thereby demanding a physical response! The stressors of today are far more subtle and our sophisticated world demands at least an outward appearance of calm control rather than a punch in the nose — even when that just might be appropriate!

All of these factors create a phenomenon first labeled by Hans Selye in 1946 as "Stress." It is "the response of our body to any change, demand, pressure or threat from outside. The aim of the stress response is to bring the agitated or disturbed body back to normal and to enable it to protect itself from the external situation."[6]

To put it all in layperson's language . . . a threat triggers defense juices which get all charged up but have no place to go. They are, therefore, absorbed. Stress management then becomes a necessity to alter the stress response so the juices don't begin eating holes in our insides!

Bear with me a few moments while I share the effects of stress on a person:[7]

1. <u>Physical Effects</u>: Elevated blood and urine catecholamines and corticosteroids; increased blood glucose, heart rate, and blood pressure; shallow, difficult breathing. Numbness, tingling and coldness of extremities; queasy stomach; tight muscles; back and head pain; dry mouth and sweating. Over time these physical responses cause breakdown of vital organs, and serious chronic disease.

2. Emotional Effects: Anxiety, anger, boredom, depression, fatigue, irritability, moodiness, tension, nervousness, self-hate, worry.

3. Mental Effects: Difficulty concentrating, poor task performance, defensiveness, focus on details, sleepiness, mental blocks.

4. Behavioral Effects: Drug use, alcoholism, smoking, over eating, loss of appetite, impulsive or agressive outbursts, accident proneness, blaming others, withdrawal or isolation.

5. Organizational Effects: Job burnout, low morale, absenteeism, poor performance, high turnover, job dissatisfaction, lawsuits, high use of health facilities, accidents, poor working relationships.

In other words, a person suffering the effects of long term stress can end up being an ill, angry, defensive, burned out worker doing a poor job and abusing various substances. Not a pretty picture.

As I look at the stress that I accumulated over many years, I see symptoms in each category that described my response with the most notable being almost weekly bouts with illness. Obviously my highly charged "juices" were eating holes in me . . . literally!

Beyond physical effects I was also feeling tense, anxious, and constantly fatigued. In the six months before my colon finally ruptured, I had problems with mental blocks during training that added to my stress by having to mask that in front of up to 1200 people. Behaviorally I'm not surprised as I look back that overeating was part of my problem when I was home and loss of appetite was prevalant when I was traveling. To complete the picture, my work lacked satisfaction for me, and I began to exhibit some classic burnout symptoms.

One of the things that helped me understand, then begin to manage, stress more healthfully was the understanding that stress comes in a three step process:

1. Stressors — (pressures, changes, demands, etc.) then . . .

2. Interpretation — (how we label the stressor through our psychological filters of expectations, beliefs, conditioning, anticipation, self-perceptions, etc.) and finally . . .

3. Our Personal, Stress Response — (arousal, fight, flight or cope)

By understanding this progression of steps, I was able to identify those points at which I could actively intervene to direct myself to more productive and appropriate responses.

It was also helpful to understand that although we have millions of ways to trigger our stress response and "turn on" our juices, we have only a few ways to turn them "off":

1. Direct, physical action (fight or flight).

2. Actively responding to a situation or by physically exercising the stress from the body.

3. Quiet forms of relaxation to activate the relaxation response.

4. Renegotiate the situation so it is no longer stressful.

Problems arise, as they did with me, when stress tension builds up due to unrelieved stress within our bodies. Jaffee and Scott tell us, "Tension is the residue that is left when we feel we cannot do something about the stress we are under, when we fail to do something about it, or when we deny its existance and mask the signs of stress. Over time, tension signals that our body has worn down, and illness is the final result."[8]

As I've studied the stress syndrome I also realized that there was another hidden stressor that I was not factoring in as such . . . the stress that comes from positive things happening in my life (called "eustress" as opposed to "distress"). It was a revelation to find out that when good things happen to people this also brings pressure and stress (job promotion, acclaim, more responsibilities, more money, new family member, etc.)

In retrospect I now realize that I was making a mistake I find common to people in the helping professions . . . the lack of transfer of high skills in management of others to self management. Obviously I found it easier to manage the efforts of 30,000 volunteers and 100,000 event participants than to effectively manage Sue Vineyard.

Under repeated pressure I had chosen to take a path of denial and avoidance leading to stress which caused illness. The better choice, and one I am now trying to retrain myself to adopt, is a creative path employing self-awareness and exploration leading to peak performance and wholistic health through self-renewal and management.

COPING WITH STRESS . . .

After focusing for such a long time on stress symptoms, I think it is time to look at ways to cope with stress. Some suggestions to consider which are detailed more completely in the suggested readings on the subject are:

1. Set realistic goals.
2. Do same things differently for variety
3. Get away . . . short or long breaks
4. Try to take things less personally
5. Focus on the positive
6. Be realistic about yourself . . . we cannot be all things to all people.
7. Rest and relax. (Whatever it takes!) Separate work and home life in your mind and have a transition or neutral zone between the two (favorite music in car going home, hot tub, etc.)
8. Establish a personal life or your own set of ways to prevent enroachment of work in private life. (I close my home office door, turn on my business answering machine in evenings, and weekends etc.)
9. Identify and pursue most relaxing leisure activities
10. Identify sources of personal strength and pursue (faith, solid relationshipc, etc.)
11. Change jobs (if all else fails!)

Getting help . . . Options . . .

1. <u>Colleagues</u> can offer immediate help, comfort, insight, comparisons, humor and escape. This may be just what you need!

2. <u>Professional help</u> may be needed by many to work their way out from under the burnout load. Trained counselors are available and should be tapped un-reluctantly to help regain balance. It may be most helpful to choose someone with whom you do not have any other agenda so it does not intrude. Ask trusted others around you for recommendations. Choosing the right professional for you is critical and it may take a few false starts before you connect with a "match" for your needs.

Improving your work situation . . .

1. *Identify goals and roles* — Who does what, when, and how are assignments interrelated?
2. *Delegate* — Come on, you can't do it all!
3. *Modify client contact* — Find creative ways to change contacts: no calls on week-ends, less work appointments, different setting, shorter consultations (or longer, whichever offers relief),

written information rather than repeating same standard replies over and over (addresses, meetings, etc.).

4. *Line up expectations with reality* — A good dose of common sense here please!
5. *Identify dependent clients and/or co-workers* and find ways to turn them elsewhere — Help them be more independent. Rid yourself of toxic relationships.
6. *Limit job spillover* to other parts of life.
7. *Take breaks* — Close the door, turn off phone, take a walk, listen to music, etc.
8. *Ask for and get help* — That's a sign of strength and maturity, NOT weakness!

Early Warning Signs of Burnout and Stress . . .

1. Listen to warnings of friends and colleagues — they usually see it first!
2. Mood changes
3. Attitude changes
4. Behavior patterns change
5. Irritability
6. Having to do work over
7. Feelings of unproductivity
8. Sense of weariness but difficulty sleeping
9. Gnawing feelings of powerlessness

Techniques for Stress Management (Burnout) . . .

There are many books written on stress/burnout management techniques, and I will not go into great descriptive detail on each, leaving you instead with a list you can add to and a bibliography of books that describe each in detail:

1. Deep muscle relaxation drill
2. Mental relaxation
3. Imagery training
4. Instant relaxation
5. Exercise
6. Hot tub or jacuzzi
7. Full body massage
8. Hobbies or diversions
9. Sharing with others
10. Meditation and/or prayer
11. Biofeedback

12. Self-hypnosis
13. Professional help
14. Journaling
15. Humor!

STRESS ... HOW DO WE CHANGE?

This book has an entire chapter devoted to Change ... but in it I am basically focusing on changes that effect you, not changes you choose to make in your life.

In trying to change my response to stressors and subsequent tension, I have come up with a process that hopefully will prevent further damage. Let me share it with you for your own adaptation and use:

1. I'm not trying to change everything all at once. I prioritize what I want to change and work on them one at a time ... (cut down on travel, train with others, etc.)

2. I have set specific goals ... very few training dates a year, only major conferences; upgrade the newsletter I write; build a product and service line in the company I co-founded with Steve McCurley; run a trainer assessment conference with Marlene Wilson once a year; take one week off with Marlene each year (cleverly titled our "Do-Nothing Week!") etc.

3. Assess constantly where I am by recording stressors as they arise.

4. Build in a reward system by identifying what is rewarding and then partaking of that golden carrot when appropriate.

5. I continue to tap true support people (having now clearly identified them) and plan contacts ... rooming with a dear friend at a conference in Florida, spending five weeks with Marlene Wilson each year (four in training, one in pure fun), meeting twice a year with three soulmates, four meetings with my business partner to keep our company on course, and having many planned and spontaneous encounters with local friends.

6. I've given up trying to be perfect. Only one person really ever was and look what happened to Him! I'm being careful not to write my plan in ink, so I can't be trapped by it ... flexibility is the order of the day, thank you.

7. I am using relaxation techniques . . . some more successfully than others, I admit, but I'm learning, and if ever I can find a good Registered Massage Therapist in my area, I should be in great shape!

8. I'm watching my attitude, believing that it is a critical factor . . . I'll allow myself an occasional blue or negative thought but not let it be a habit. I am trying to positively reinforce myself. This has been a challenge when my body does not respond healthfully, as I seem to slip into a "now what?" attitude that could (if unchecked) become a self-fulfilling prophecy.

9. I'm working to rely more heavily on my spiritual dimension . . . finding ways to refresh, praying more, reading more uplifting books and spiritual thoughts, discussing this facet of my life with others I feel are ahead of me in spiritual strength, and possibly finding a new spiritual home and mentor.

10. I'm being careful to listen and respond more carefully to my body signals . . . many of which are new to me. This has been quite an undertaking, as my pattern was to put off response indefinately or to a more "convenient" time. Now, like E.F. Hutton, when my body speaks, I listen!

11. I am continuing to look for ways to have fun and to play. I deeply believe in the power of laughter . . . the giggle surely is mightier than the groan!

I'd like to tell you this plan of attack on my stress responders is 100% sure-fire, fail-safe, but it's probably not and will require adjustment, revision, and additions to make it work for me. The real point is, however, that I have a plan at all and am actively working at staying and keeping healthy . . . physically, emotionally, mentally, spiritually, and relationally.

Won't you join me?

Seven Causes of Stress . . .

In an article entitled "Straight Talk About Stress" by Robert A. Jud[9] which appeared in a 1985 March/April issue of the Executive Female, the author lists seven common causes of stress in individuals.

Jud, who has been offering consulting services in adult learning areas for many years, remarked on both negative and positive stress

. . . the former being harmful to health and welfare, the latter being exhilarating and challenging.

As caregivers who work in organizations, we can benefit from looking closely at these seven areas, assessing how each affects us and identifying our responses to each type of stressor we must deal with.

The seven areas of common stresses are:

1. *Change* . . . I've devoted a whole chapter to this subject, and Jud simply reaffirms my belief that when we find change in routines, habits and rhythms in our life, we feel off balance and need time to readjust. This is true even when the change is positive, such as a promotion, the holidays, or a vacation.

2. *Expectations* . . . when expectations of others or yourself do not match reality. Victor Vroom detailed this in his Theory of Expectancy, warning us of upheaval when reality and expectations don't mesh. Jud quotes MIT psychologist Dean Ornish who says, "In my judgement, the greatest stressor of all is the mismatch of who and where I am and who and where I think I ought to be."

3. *Perfectionism* . . . as caregivers and those in the business of helping others, we frequently fall into the trap of wanting all our efforts to be successful. The failure of our efforts on behalf of even one client, student, patient, volunteer, worker, etc. is more than we can bear, causing us to be trapped in our own web of oughts and shoulds as it relates to our behavior.

4. *Inability to set limits* . . . this is where we try to be all things to all people . . . counselor, mentor, priest, friend, teacher, rescuer, fixer, etc. etc. It is almost an occupational hazzard with caregivers and one with dire consequences. It's the super woman or man image coming home to roost!

5. *Conflict and confrontation* . . . because we need the approval of others, we frequently cannot see conflict as a constructive way to clear the air. Instead we see it as destructive or as an attack, and we'll twist ourselves out of shape to avoid it, including games-playing, suppression of true feelings, and a whole lot of gunny-sacking of anger and resentment. This again, is typical of caregivers who seem to have a self-image of peacemaker, always smiling and making things right. Somehow, conflict seems out of place in this picture and is avoided at all costs, resulting in stress to oneself and the organization.

6. *Type A behavior* . . . first described by Meyer Friedman and Ray Rosenman, this is the pedal to the metal, panic driven person who goes at everything in racing gear . . . constantly risking, reaching for the next plateau and rarely, if ever, stopping to find steady footing or comfort. For this kind of person, life is a constant race and struggle, needing to accomplish more and more in less and less time.

7. *Fear of ambiguity* . . . an excessive need for control (often labeled as Type B personality). A desire and need to have everything neat and orderly, totally predictable and clear . . . a rare commodity in our world of human services where no case or project is ever exactly the same because of the human factors involved.

It is critical for us to look at stress in our life from this suggested perspective so that we might see its effect on us, for either good or bad. Stress is really our response to events that happen around us and our reaction to them. Knowing simply if we fit in the pattern of Type A (Go! Go! Go!) or Type B (Control, control, control) is helpful in assessing our potential stress responses.

I believe that the more ways we have of looking at ourselves honestly and the more information we have on the critical dimension of stress, the more prepared we will be as we cope with life and its surprises.

YOUR STRESS BAGGAGE LIMIT . . .

For the last 12 years I have spent a good portion of my time on various airplanes; some are huge, some have more seats in them than our local theater. Others are small and cramped and even when full don't offer enough space for a complete football team.

This latter, pint-sized variety is my least favorite, and when I first began to cut down on my travel schedule, they afforded me a great excuse to turn down dates in remote areas.

My reasons for disliking small aircraft are many, but always highlighted by one particularly unnerving requirement — that of being asked to get on a scale with your luggage to "weigh in." True, I am a wee bit sensitive that my own weight does not match my driver's license claim, but my real consternation comes from wondering what would happen if the scale was malfunctioning and we took off a pound or two "overweight."

The exercise of "weighing in" and calculating all the cumulative baggage you must carry has a good lesson for us as we examine our own "stress baggage."

By that phrase I refer to all of the stressors we carry with us each day — some long term (like chronic illness) and others, short term (like a flooded basement).

As I look back over the years of my own stress build up, I recognize that I was not really aware of my own baggage and therefore piled on more without ever "weighing in" to see what its cumulative effect might be.

The heaviest baggage I was carrying but denying is the long term effect of having a handicapped child. He would resent that term, but I have no better word to use. "Disabled" is worse and "challenged" sounds like something out of Pollyanna.

Born with a severe learning disability that created a million-character alphabet and made calculation and concepts as clear as hieroglyphics on a cave wall, our eldest son struggled with school and systems and graphic learning as a child wrestling with a bear.

Until his entry into school, the handicap was hidden to the world, masked behind a higher than average IQ, a quick wit and charming face framed by golden hair and bright blue eyes.

I can recall with intense pain the phone call from his first grade teacher, herself the parent of a learning disabled child, as she told me gently but straightforwardly, "your son has a handicap."

Her call began a long succession of trips to doctors, neurologists, psychologists, special education teachers and diagnosticians that ended in special schooling, enormous debt and a pattern of two steps forward, one step back for a dozen years and more.

My husband and I were tossed from emotional pillar to post by "professionals" who exclaimed everything from "Forget him, you have another son!" to "He has a brilliant mind if only you find a way to develop it" and of course, the ever present falsehood: "Oh, ignore it — he'll grow out of it!"

If you ever want to test your mettle as a parent, have someone tell you you have a handicapped child. That realization caused my adrenelin to get stuck on "high" as I fought for his special education, self-confidence and every success I could put in his path. I took on a school system that didn't want to provide proper education (they finally did), a town without a learning disabled parental support group (established within four months), psychologists with pat answers that weren't really applicable (they disappeared, mumbling, into the sunset), and a verbally abusive teacher who would stand our son up in front of his fourth grade class and point out his deficiencies to "embarrass him into learning" (fired, thank you).

I'd like to tell you all this has a Hollywood ending, with our son now a famous brain surgeon, but life isn't that well scripted, and

I'm simply thrilled that he seems content and happy today with new-found skills in remodeling homes. I'm also experienced enough to know that tomorrow might bring a different story in the continuing pattern of two steps forward, one step back.

Life has been painful for him, and through the years my heaviest concentration and investment was on trying to ease this pain, to let him experience some, but not all, of the hard knocks and to, above all, let him know how much I loved him and how OK he was with me.

Throughout all this effort directed at helping him, I shoved to the background of my mind the real pain I felt at the circumstances of his life.

I denied the reality that the son I thought I had for six years ("if he chooses he can be President — anything is possible and open to him!") had evaporated and in his place was a child with limitations.

That statement probably makes some readers angry — as if I thought he was the less for his handicap. That interpretation would not only be inaccurate but unfair. Parents of handicapped children have one great need in common — the acceptance of what is and the letting go of what cannot be.

To hope for a future as an air-ground controller for a blind child is unrealistic. To insist that a child born with cerebral palsy be a famous ballet dancer "if only they try hard enough" is to set up a life of frustration, and to impose an unrealistic goal for a child with a severe problem with discalcula (difficulty calculating) to ever be a great mathematician "if you really work at it," is to look for palm trees in the Antarctic.

The reality is of course that we all have limitations, but those imposed on the handicapped are often greater and more far reaching than on the average person. Our need is to accept things we cannot change while recognizing opportunities to change the things we can.

My own acceptance of our son's limitations was slow to come, but did manifest itself eventually. What did not come until very recently, was a realization of the toll his handicap had taken on me and the constant stress baggage it caused me to carry in life.

Many of us have long term stress baggage we must carry every day. It is critical for us to recognize its existence as each of us has a weight limit beyond which we cannot extend without disastrous results.

To be aware of what our "base" baggage is — and therefore how much more additional weight we can take on — is a key factor in assessing our stress load limit.

Examine the various dimensions of your life. Are there constant stressors that are simply a part of your every day load? Chronic illness, a handicapped child, poor health of a loved one, overwhelming debt, a hereditary time bomb (I have a friend whose mother and aunt died of Huntington's Chorea — St. Vitus Dance — and therefore has a 50-50 chance of having the same affliction in middle age), an unhappy marriage, estrangement from family, a hated job, poverty, etc. etc. All can be the cause for a basic heavy stress load to which little else must be added to have our physical, emotional, mental or spiritual dimension read "TILT!"

I have come to learn that there are times when I can absorb more stress than others. While recuperating from the first surgery for the colostomy, I discovered, much to my schagrin, that I found even the most elementary decisions too stressful to handle.

When a friend called and began to share a stress with me, I had to cut her off, explaining that I was simply in no shape to take on any more stress than what I was already handling. I was too close to "overload."

I believe it is important to constantly assess your stress-load, evaluating how heavy or light it is.

At "light" times I urge you to tackle those projects and challenges that you've set aside and correctly identified as ones that will produce stress. At times of heavy stress loads, I urge you to put those same projects and challenges off and not feel guilty at doing so. (Better to do something right at a later time than wrong immediately!)

What is your stress load? What are the "givens" you must deal with daily? What is their cummulative effect? How much more can you take on? When more stress is imposed, what other stresses can you shed?

If there were such a thing as a stress scale, how much would you weigh? And what is the upperlimit before overweight occurs? (See Holmes-Rahe Test, page 35).

And the real bottom-line question — with the stress weight you carry, can you really fly safely and get to your destination?

GUILT ... THE ENEMY WITHIN ...

In his book, <u>When Bad Things Happen To Good People</u>[10] Harold Kushner continually comes back to the theme of unnecessary guilt that people feel when something goes wrong in their lives or the lives of those around them.

He shares story after story of people who add to the stresses already in their life by feeling that bad circumstances around them are somehow their fault. "If only" and "I should or should not have" statements frame agonized people's feelings, thus doubling pain unnecessarily.

In talking and working with helping professionals, I hear an over abundance of "If only," "Should," and "Ought" statements surrounding their work, clients, co-workers, family, friends, etc.

Somehow we, who have such high ideals about helping to make this world a better place, begin to take responsibility for everyone and everything around us. When life events and relationships go awry due to the fact that it is an imperfect world, we can often take on feelings of guilt that are really quite irrational.

In my last two years with the charity I spoke of earlier, I was angry, frustrated, and disillusioned with disabling management practices. I suffered the added and unnecessary burden of feeling guilty that I couldn't "make everything work".

When, after submitting a proposal for a new fundraising idea three times and having it rejected, first because it was single spaced, second because its margins were too narrow, and third because it was then "too long," I felt guilt at my own anger and inability to get across an idea I felt would help our clients.

I said things to myself such as, "I should be able to find ways to get my ideas across without offending my supervisor," "I ought to be bigger than the anger I feel," "I shouldn't be frustrated by the lack of focus on the needs of the clients" and "If only I'd waited until my boss was in a better mood."

All of these feelings were guilt trips I was laying on myself that put the blame on me for the idea not being considered. In truth, the probem lay wih my supervisor and the games he was playing with me. Sadly, my own preoccupation with my guilt and frustration denied me the perspective I needed to deal with his classic passive-aggressive behavior and manipulation.

As I've shared that story in several training sessions (to help people uncover what a problem is and what it is not), I've had many people share other, similar stories where they somehow felt responsible, and subsequently guilty, for rotten things being done to them!

We seem to recognize unnecessary guilt in others: the children of divorced parents who blame themself for the breakup; the parent who loses a child to an accident and blames themself for not watching them more closely; an adult who feels they were the cause of their elderly parents death because they put them in a nursing home.

When confronted with such people, we are quick to counsel them about their feelings of total responsibility for events in the lives of loved ones.

At the same time however, helping professionals can feel guilty about things that are going wrong around them, feeling that somehow they are responsible and should make it "right."

65

One of the most common guilt trips I run into is the "I should be able to work with _____, after all, we're all here for the same high purpose . . . to help others." Sometimes the focus is on working with another person, at other times it can be rules and regulations, and still other times, limitations that are forced on us.

In any of these cases, we feel we should be more patient, accepting, understanding, forgiving, tolerant or whatever to make the situation workable for the greater cause.

Unfortunately this unrealistic judgment of ourselves sets up a chain reaction of shoulds, oughts, self-directed disappointment, denial of real feelings, guilt and clouded issues. Instead of conflict resolution it leads to dual conflicts — that between ourselves and others and that raging within ourselves, against ourselves!

The bare truth of the matter is that although we often enter into our work to save the world with an expectation that everyone we meet is there for the same high purpose, we need to quickly become more realistic about our efforts and those around us.

The first reality is that we can't save everyone — there are too many of "them" and some don't want to be saved!

As a trainer I had to quickly come to realize that not everyone who came to my training sessions really wanted to be taught. For some, the purpose for coming to hear me, was to negate what I was proposing.

I can recall one middle-aged manager of a national charity that fought me every step of the way during a day-long session on positive, enabling volunteer management. He did everything to disrupt the training, discredit my message, and even me personally.

In talking with embarrassed subordinates and his supervisor over lunch, I found that he was known for his tyrannical management of both paid and unpaid staff that caused people to continually leave his regional office.

He had been given a mandate to change his style "or else," and he was insisting that any new management style (such as the one I was teaching) simply wouldn't work. His purpose, therefore, was to shoot down what I was saying. He had come to NOT learn!

Abraham Maslow said once, "Refusal to learn is more deeply a refusal to do" and Alice Sergeant, in her book Androgynous Manager[11] shared, "Denial is the alternative to change." Both were pointing out that some people do not want to be helped (or saved, or trained, etc.) because they are comfortable where they are and fearful of change.

When I understood this I no longer felt responsible for every single person's learning in all my audiences and therefore let go of any guilt for someone's lack of learning.

Before accepting this lesson, I felt very badly if one or two people in an audience of 100 wrote a negative evaluation after one of my sessions. I agonized over the two, ignoring the 98 who valued my work, and I felt real guilt that I'd somehow "failed."

I see the same guilt weighing human service workers down, as they look at the few clients they were unable to help rather than the many they were.

The second reality, after accepting that we really can't save everyone, is to understand that not everyone we must deal with in our mission to serve others is going to be nice, good, fair, or adult. (A sign I once saw said: "If you plan to be a Princess understand you'll have to kiss a lot of toads before you find your Prince!")

Among the princes of the world there are a few toads, and we need to stop expecting that they'll somehow turn into a prince if we simply are nice, fair, understanding, and friendly enough with them.

We begin to offer excuses for the toads, saying things like: "If I just give him time, he'll come around and play fair," or "If I show her how good it can be for our clients, she'll stop blocking my efforts," or "If I could find better ways to communicate, they'll understand."

Wrong.

There are people who, for whatever reasons will always feel threatened by capable people with good, new ideas and will work to squash them. There are those who are unconsciously incompetent and will never "understand." There are those to whom their personal power and control is more important than helping clients or allowing others to grow. There are still others who have personal scores to settle and believe that they are justified by any means to do so and finally, those who only feel good by putting others down.

As much as we would like to think so, all the people working in human service, churches, education, health and welfare, charities and public service jobs are NOT well-meaning, selfless, committed, well-balanced people. Some are downright mean, selfish, misguided souls with a few bricks missing from a full load!

For those people who must work over, with, or under such people to feel guilty in their relationships with them is very unrealistic. All the kisses in the world won't turn these toads into princes!

Fortunately the toad population is very low in comparison to the princes and princesses, with a lot of people falling somewhere between the two.

As caregivers we must be realistic in our expectations of others around us, keeping ourselves healthy by rejecting unnecessary guilt when things go wrong.

As far as I know, none of us has been elected President of the World!

The third reality is often so cleverly disguised that it is hardly recognizable. That is that self-expectations in regard to a reputation can be deadly.

I call it the "Living up to my own press clipping" or "Mother-superior" syndrome! And I've been in a position to see several people succomb to it.

The scenario is such that a person builds a reputation as a wise, caring, sympathetic, "I'll help you" being. Others are attracted to the person and feel warm toward them, offering much praise and honor for their wonderful nature and wise ways.

Their reputation grows as people who have been helped tell others of their skills and even suggest they get in touch with this wonderful person to help THEM with their problems.

Soon the line is long at the door of the wonderperson, with people alternately asking for help and praising their kindness. A few even try to cannonize them, claiming they've produced miracles.

For wonderperson, it feels good to help so many, to be appreciated, to make a difference in the lives of others, etc. Their ego glows as time passes and more examples of positive results from their requested intervention mounts along with their reputation and demands for help.

While this is going on, wonderperson comes to accept a self-image as all-caring, a listener, and a helper of others. At a deeper, unconscious level, there is a rejection of opposite qualities so they begin to form a list of what they are "not". In case you've never confronted your own thoughts on what you say you are "not," think back to the times you felt most wounded, most wronged, and the most defensive. I'll bet someone accused you of something you said you were 'not!"

Subliminally, wonderperson begins to feed themselves with messages such as "I am never uncaring," "I am not a poor listener," "I do not abandon people when they need help," "I am not unwise."

Suddenly, they find themselves in the position of trying to help everyone because they feel guilty about not doing so. They resist any feelings of not helping others because they have convinced themselves that being a non-helper is abhorrent.

Several trainers I know have developed such reputations for being willing to listen and "fix" peoples' woes, (personal or organizational) that much of their energies go into therapy sessions after hours, draining their strength for the work they were hired to do and their personal, wholistic health. It is obvious that guilt prevents them from walking away from the idea of helping everyone.

I fell into this category for several years as a trainer, when I agreed to listen to everyone's problems, sometimes until two in the morning! Every coffee break, meal and free minute were taken in counseling others. I felt good in helping others sort out their problems, and it afforded me an opportunity to use my own gifts.

Trips that were scheduled to encompass six hours of training expanded beyond that during eight to ten more hours of counseling and problem solving. Even though satisfied at the day's end for helping, I still had to contend with being physiclly, mentally, and emotionally exhausted.

I rejected saying "no" to others out of guilt ("who am I to not share my gifts when people need them?") and because I'd become comfortable and even warmed by my reputation as an all-wise, sympathetic person who could help anyone through anything.

It is critical that we learn, as Moses did in the Old Testament when he was reprimanded by his father-in-law for trying to deal with eveyone's problems, that we must be a steward of our own strength and recognize our own limitations.

We need to distinguish between the fantasies that can develop around a reputation for perfection and the reality of our own humanity and its resultant needs to say "no" to others' demands so we can say "yes" to our own.

We must reject guilt about saying no and run the risk of tarnishing the wonderperson reputation. Lastly we need to look realistically at our own self-expectations to see how damaging they might be to our wholistic health.

Guilt is a subtle adversary — it shows its face through "shoulds" and "oughts" and "if only" statements we hear ourselves make. It grinds away at all dimensions of our being and twists us into unnecessary pain and agony. It drains us; causes us to lose sight of reality and puts us out of touch with the messages our body and soul send out.

In short, it is an enemy within.

CAREGIVERS AS CARE TAKERS:
WE'RE TERRIBLE AT IT! . . .

A paradox seems to exist for those people who are best at caring for others in that when caregivers have needs in their own lives, they are terrible at accepting help. Or to put it simply: "People who are best at giving help are worst at accepting it."

A friend and Pastor who recently suffered a stroke is struggling with being the recipient of help. He is especially having difficulty in expressing what is and is not helpful.

A manager of volunteer services, so used to assisting others, vehemently rejects even the suggestion that she accept assistance in her battle against an arthritic condition.

A counselor to many pretends she's "fine" when she's really emotionally drained, for fear of seeming less than "OK."

In each case, I see caregivers struggling with a reverse role as "care-takers" or "care-needers."

A friend of mine, Jean Parker, who is a nurse and ostomy specialist at Hinsdale Hospital here in Illinois, and I recently discussed how terrible medical personnel are as patients, how reluctant social workers are to seek guidance, and how infrequently caregivers such as herself express their own needs or accept unsolicited help.

One of the new found joys in my own life is willingness to be open to others about what I need and don't need and to accept help from others who can support me in my life's journey.

In the section on relationships I stress the critical importance of supportive interactions with others; to identify soul mates and those who celebrate your successes; to eliminate toxic relationships or those for which you hold unrealistic expectations, etc.

Having identified your caregivers is only the first step, however. When the needs arise the next step must be taken — to accept their help when offered and to ask for it when it's needed.

I find an inordinate amount of embarrassment and anxiety in caregivers when they must accept help from others. Somehow they seem to feel it weakens them, and they are uncomfortable with reversed roles of needing rather than giving.

I've even experienced people who become very angry at the notion that they need help. I can recall a time several years ago when I found myself reacting with anger and frustration when I physically needed assistance. Somehow I felt the less for my need — weaker, less in control, less valuable.

When I came to grips with the fact that I had developed an always-in-control self image and had confused my works with my worth, I was able to accept help from others more comfortably. Instead of feeling any the lesser for needing help I felt the richer, as I grew closer to soul mates and friends who had a chance to express their love and concern for me in tangible ways.

I began to see how my pride and sense of independence had stopped me from calling out for help far beyond when I first needed it. And most beautifully, I found a deeper awareness of how to help others by accepting help from others.

I also learned to sort out those people who truly could be counted on for help and those who could not (the "fair weather" friends my Grandmother used to describe), and though painful, it was a valuable sorting.

Somehow caregivers become so engrained in their helping roles, seeing those helped as on the other side of the coin, they have trouble switching roles comfortably and with grace. We have trouble saying "I need" while still finding it second nature to say "Let me help."

When trouble comes and you find yourself in need of help, it may be useful to enter into a quick "neutral zone" to enable you to make the transition from "caregiver" to "care-taker."

WORTH AND WORK ... AND BIG RED FLAGS! ...

My paternal Grandfather was the master mechanic on the Elgin, Joliet and Eastern Railroad out of Joliet, Illinois, and I delighted in his sharing stories from the "yard" regarding work he was doing there.

I can recall his telling me that whenever something was found to be amiss with the engines, a red flag was placed on the site to signal a need for him to repair the damage.

I have often thought how wonderfully easy it would be for us as human beings if we could see red flags marking those places within that require attention and possible repair.

One such area within me, that was spotted by one very close to me, was a confusion that I had allowed to develop of my worth and my work ... mixing up my value as an individual and my value as a trainer, author, and consultant.

As I examined this confusion in myself, I recognized it as a rather common problem among people who care for and serve others. So many people I talk with, when asked to describe themselves, tell me of the work they do ... an agency director, a nurse, a Pastor, a manager, etc. For some, it is almost impossible to think of themselves in any other way than through their work and I feel a gnawing concern that they too may have confused these two distinct things.

When we speak of the worth of an individual we are talking about their essence ... their personality and values, faith and beliefs, relationships and caring, responses and feelings. When we are talking about work, we are talking about actions, a job and assignments. The two are very different, though they are intertwined.

I ache for the volunteer administrator in Iowa who was dispondent over having missed four days of work due to the flu ... "whatever will my volunteers think of me?" she shared. In California I talked with a Pastor who was running himself ragged, over-booking his schedule so that he had little time for his family and no time for himself, but continued on convinced that 'this is the only way I know to really make a difference in my parish." Last there was the woman in North Carolina who confided that she had gone to work several times when she was seriously ill because, "I don't want people to think I'm a shirker!"

In each case, through continued conversation with the above people, it became clear to me that they had totally overlaid the definitions of worth and work in their minds to the point that they were one and the same. Each was saying that doing less work made them less valuable to others and that their contributions were measured by the volume of what they did rather than its quality or their own personal value as a whole.

Having walked in those moccasins, I could understand their confusion, and how easy it is for caregivers to get to that point. So much of what we do is quantified . . . how many clients? how many volunteers? What's the cost? How much time did you spend? etc . . . that we can begin to think only in numbers rather than overall effect.

As one who is evaluated every time I work (trainers have that curse/joy!), I slid easily into believing that the evaluations on my work were an evaluation on me as a person, especially since so many people personalize their comments on a training event . . . "I think you're great or awful" rather than "I think the training was great or awful". It was an easy next step to take to feel that by doing more training and saying yes to more peoples' demands that I was therefore more valuable, and conversely, that doing less made me less so.

When I was confronted with physical problems that demanded a lessening of my schedule, a raging battle was begun within me, as I fought the feeling of being less valuable to the people around me because I could not fill all their needs. Unfortunately, no one was around to place a red flag on this inappropriate response in its early stage to warn that it needed "repair," so I suffered under his confusion for several years before one of my soul mates pointed it out to me.

When she did, I immediately felt a lifting of my spirits and a great light bulb went off somehwere in my soul, as I separated the two portions of Sue Vineyard for once and for always.

In my work, it had remarkable results . . . lifting off the guilt I had felt if I said "no" to too many requests for piggybacking, meetings morning, noon and night and "off" hours demands for my ear and "fixit" salve. I was able to schedule in line with realistic understanding of my stamina; I was able to say no when requests went beyond reasonable demands, and I could remove a lot of "oughts" and "shoulds" from my internal self-talk.

In my personal life, it had fascinating repercussions, as I had tried to be an ever ready friend, making sure sick friends had a casserole, that I responded to every possible request for my energies, etc. Instead,

72

I did what I could to be supportive, but without feeling I had to meet every need or play total servant when things were amiss in friend's lives. As a consequence, I lost a friend or two, who could not adjust to anything less than a totally serving Sue Vineyard. Though painful, I feel that was a good sorting out period as I identified those who liked me for me and those who liked me for what I did.

In counseling others who are under stress, I try to probe gently at their clarity of themselves as a person and themselves as a worker, to see if there is any confusion in this area. Typcially, I find some confusion in caregivers as they feel guilty at what they have not done and somehow "bad" for not doing it.

This problem is not an uncommon one among the general population. Recently I heard about an engineer who, upon losing his job, sank into a deep depression, became physically ill and lethargic. He refused counseling; he interpreted that as not only worthless but weak, as well. Tragically his eventual decision was suicide as he could never separate his worth as an indivdual from that of his not being able to be an engineer.

Others, when faced with the cessation of a particular job chose a different path, so that the newly blind artist became a teacher; the quadrapelegic nurse became a writer and creator of games, and the actor who lost his voice box became a counselor to others with the same trauma and a champion for the handicapped.

In each case, these people saw that they were much more than any particular line of work. They knew their worth lay in their essence, not their job.

As you assess your wholistic health and look for red flags in your stress load, examine this area of worth and work . . . do they feel like one and the same? Can you distinguish between the "doer" that is you and the real person that is you? Can you see options of other work than what you are now doing that would alter what you do but not who you are inside? Do you understand that the people who truly love, like, and respect you are interested in you as a person and a relationship in their life, and what you do is not the main consideration? Can you accept the idea that successful living is qualitative and not only quantitative?

By confusing worth and work, we are really taking only the short term view of life. The long term view tells us that going to work when we are ill can lead to serious health problems; that guilt over what we cannot do is destructive, and that stretching ourselves too thin is eventually going to catch up with us.

The people who mean the most to us would be the people who would be most forceful in trying to get these messages across. Often it is one of them who must first plant the red flag on this confusion, demanding that we repair our thinking.

As several dear friends shared with me recently, "We don't care if you clerk at the dimestore, as long as you are around to share our lives with us!".

As workers and care givers who constantly "do" things for others, we need to constantly separate worth and work in our minds. We must not attach our own personal value to the jobs we do, lest we equate any change or lessening of our work to a lesser worth as a person.

Each person is valuable for what they are, how they relate to others, what gifts they share in life, their personalities and values and the essence that makes up "them." Their works, though valuable, do not tell the whole story, and are not, to the people who mean the most to them, the measure of their worth.

If you find yourself disagreeing with this statement or even being uncomfortable with it, I might suggest placing a big red flag on your reaction.

KEEPING SCORE . . .

In her wonderful book Gifts of Grace[12] Mary Schramm quotes a parable by Ann Herbert on keeping score:

> "In the beginning God didn't make just one or two people; he made a bunch of us. Because he wanted us to have a lot of fun and he said you can't really have fun unless there's a whole gang of you. So he put us all in this sort of playground park place called Eden and told us to enjoy.
>
> At first we did have fun just like he expected. We played all the time. We rolled down the hills, waded in the streams, climbed the trees, swung on the vines, ran in the meadows, frolicked in the woods, hid in the forest, and acted silly. We laughed a lot.
>
> Then one day this snake told us that we weren't having real fun because we weren't keeping score. Back then, we didn't know what score was. When he explained it, we still couldn't see the fun. But he said that we should give an apple to the person who was best at playing and we'd never know who was best unless we kept score. We could all see the fun of that. We were all sure we were best.

It was different after that. We yelled a lot. We had to make up new scoring rules for most of the games we played. Other games, like frolicking, we stopped playing because they were too hard to score. By the time God found out about our new fun, we were spending about forty-five minutes a day in actual playing and the rest of the time working out the score. God was wroth about that — very, very wroth.

He said we couldn't use his garden anymore because we weren't having any fun. We said we were having lots of fun and we were. He shouldn't have got upset just because it wasn't exactly the kind of fun he had in mind.

He wouldn't listen. He kicked us out and said we couldn't come back until we stopped keeping score. To rub it in (to get our attention, he said), he told us we were all going to die anyway and our scores wouldn't mean anything.

He was wrong. My cumulative all-game score is now 16,548 and that means a lot to me. If I can raise it to 20,000 before I die I'll know I've accomplished something. Even if I can't my life has a great deal of meaning because I've taught my children to score high and they'll all be able to reach 20,000 or even 30,000 I know.

Really, it was life in Eden that didn't mean anything. Fun is great in its place, but without scoring there's no reason for it. God has a very superficial view of life and I'm glad my children are being raised away from his influence. We were lucky to get out. We're all very grateful to the snake."

When I first read this, I was working on a training seminar for recognition, and I found it applicable to the negative definition of recognition which only rewards quantity not quality.

Too frequently we see volunteer programs, human service groups, schools, churches, governmental departments etc. keeping a tally sheet that shows hours, days or years of service but does not go beyond, to the depth of people's commitment, service, and involvement.

As people in the helping professions, we are asked to quantify much of what we do — clients served, hours worked, patient numbers, pupil ratio etc., and it is easy to fall into a mind set of keeping score.

Since this isn't a book on management I'll leave to other works my thoughts on how destructful and misleading it can be for an organization to simply keep numerical score cards on people and miss the real importance found in the quality of work done. As this is, however, a book on the management of you I would like to look at the pitfalls we can encounter when evaluating ourself on numbers alone and the real dangers inherent in what we expect when others evaluate us.

Let me share several examples of experiences where the scorekeeping has become a handicap.

A friend of mine recently came back from a three week trip where he proudly announced he'd survived 18 consultations and training dates. When I asked him how they went he stated honestly, "The first five went well, after that it was all a blur". In this instance, scorekeeping (of the number of jobs one can accomplish in a span of time) had become the goal and the quantity of work outshadowed the quality.

Steve McCurley and I, who have a partnership of training, consulting, marketing, and publishing, set out a simple goal at the outset of our work together — the quality of what we offer is more important than the quantity. Keeping this in mind we each book ourselves only to the point that we feel we can deliver a good product. This is different for each of us to be sure, but each of us sets our own limit that defines the perimeter of our best quality. To venture beyond this limit is, we feel, to invite disaster.

Workers in human service must beware of exceeding their own personal and professional perimeters of quality and resist the temptation to simply do more, faster each year and label that "progress." In truth it is usually just score keeping.

After being ill and knowing I must reduce the number of training dates I accept each year, I was confronted with my own "score keeping" attitudes to make sure I would not feel any sense of failure because I would be doing less workshops.

Fortunately I found I could feel good about reducing my numbers even drastically because I knew that by having fewer on my calendar I could give more attention, energy and thus quality to each.

It is important to examine your score keeping goals to see that they are appropriate, long ranged and a stimulant to positivity in your life — a help not a hinderance.

Another view of score keeping came in dealing with a health care worker recently who expressed deep resentment toward her institution for not recognizing a milestone (ten years) in her work with them. She was angry at her boss, co-workers, and the institution in general. As she vented her frustration I heard her use "scoring" words over and over: "After all the hours I've tallied you'd think . . .," "As I add up these last ten years I see . . .," All my work must count for nothing from the way they treat me . . . ," "I produce more work than two other people combined, yet no one appreciates me!" etc. etc.

It was obvious to me that keeping score was a major part of her perception of her job and being rewarded was a high expectation of hers. When her tenth anniversary came and went without a peep, a cake, or a card she felt denied "rightful" reward.

We need to be careful if we are indeed score keepers that we recognize the painful truth that possibly no one else has our same score card on the top shelf of their mind!

When we set up expectations for others, especially tied to specific numbers and dates, we can often be let down and hurt as others fail to live up to our expectations.

We must also recognize that we may be more of a score keeper than we think. When I left the national charity as its National Director in 1979 I received a plaque thanking me for my "Five Years of Service." The plaque hangs on my wall but evokes a mixed reaction since I was with them six years. Somehow, though I do not think of myself as a score keeper, I still feel they might have gotten the number of years right!

A last example of score keeping comes from an acquaintance of mine some years ago who I swear must have had a score card on her refrigerator for each of her "friends."

When I'd run into her at meetings she'd often say, (pointedly) "Why haven't you called me? I called you last week", or "We'll look forward to spending an evening with you soon — it is your turn to have us over I believe" or "Since I took Bill and Bob for about four hours last month could you take XXX for a full eight hour day next week?"

Whew! and Goodbye!

That kind of "let's keep our scores even" kind of thinking can drive even a CPA crazy. Thank goodness she moved away — can you imagine how she'd be with a computer to keep score?

In relationships score keeping to excess cannot serve the larger goal of life-sharing very well. Please do not think I'm advocating a totally unbalanced relationship where one gives 90% the other 10% — that won't work either and is not healthy for those involved. But I am suggesting that in mature, open, giving relationships over the years, score keeping is not necessary — it will all even out eventually and even if it doesn't precisely, it will be of no real consequence.

My closest personal friends are up to 4000 miles away from my home. I suppose if you only kept a score card on how many actual hours a year we are together it might look as though I'm an under-priviledged friend. Actually it's just the opposite — the relatively few hours we have together are full of top quality relating and fun, and we make the most of our time together — not because we're keeping score, but because we're not!

As you look at drains and stresses that might be on you presently, examine the whole arena of score keeping

Is yours in proper perspective? Does it have realistic expectations in relation to others and yourself? Is it balanced? Is it obsessive? Does it account for quality?

Wholistic health can be a step closer when we avoid score keeping and instead focus on balancing.

TIME — FRIEND OR FOE? ...

I'll bet you thought I was going to quote here from Alan Larkins famous book and video <u>How To Get Control of Your Time and Your Life.</u>[13]

Wrong.

Though I feel it's an excellent tool that offers one way to organize your time, I'm going to spare you a recital of its message of prioritizing demands and instead look at time from a broader perspective. (If you feel you need a "what do I do first?" book on time management I'd suggest you read Larkin's book or the chapter on time management in Marlene Wilson"s book, <u>Survival Skills for Managers.</u>[14])

Whenever I talk with people in the helping professions about "burnout," gathering case studies as I go, I hear constant referrals to time and its constraints.

Just as the computer has become the whipping post for all errors, so has time become the catch-all "It's-not-my-fault!" excuse for unaccomplished goals.

Certainly there are occasions when an imposed timeframe <u>was</u> too short for the assigned work, but more often than not blaming time was a way to divert attention from poor planning, improper management, or a lack of skills.

Let's examine each of these three reasons for disappointment or failure both in relation to time and as the real cause of problems subsequently blamed on "time."

1. *Poor Planning and Time* — As I have specialized in helping people plan fundraiser and marketing stragegies, I have frequently had opportunities to watch people judge the time it will take them to accomplish their goals. More often than not, the biggest mistake they make is allowing too little time for too large a job.

Instead of sitting down and mapping out all of the things and efforts that must come together before a goal can be attained they superficially guess at a time length without careful study or the input of others involved.

One group, putting on a nationally advertised event, so misjudged the time it would take to put the program together, contacting speakers, getting confirmation of seminars, obtaining training descriptions, designing the schedule, etc. etc. that they were two months late in getting their major marketing piece, which described the program, to the public.

This caused a domino effect that ended with a conference half the size it could have been (thus half the revenue for the sponsoring organization!). Had they been more realistic on their time-frame and more managerially adept when they saw people falling behind in timelines, their conference could have been much larger.

I'm always amazed at messages left on my answering machine that say "We're having a conference in four weeks and want you to Keynote. Please call me back today to verify because our program needs to go to the printer by five o'clock!".

Needless to say, my travel schedule does not permit me to be in my office every day to answer such messages and quite a few people are startled to find out I can't get back to them for a day or two. (P.S. — I never take a job that indicates such poor planning — I did once at the start of my training career and it was the disaster you'd expect!)

When planning for any event, look carefully at a realistic timeline. Bring everyone into the planning stage that will be involved so you can work their time frames into yours. Then add a week or two for margin and have at it!

This will allow you to plan successfully and avoid any necessity of blaming poor old beleaguered "TIME" for any shortcomings!

2. *Improper Management and Time* — When I am asked to consult with a group or agency in management and find a lot of "time-made-me-do-it" excuses (much akin to "the-devil-made-me-do-it" declarations) I find the hair on the back of my neck standing straight up.

Usually, through further exploration of what the real problem is, I uncover poor management practices that are being camouflaged by the great time excuse.

Chief among the managerial culprits is a lack of delegation, poor job descriptions and a lack of understanding of the ultimate goal of the effort.

Too often we find people convinced that if they don't do everything it won't be done right, or people who feel that everything must be done now as it has been in the past, even if that "past" is 100 years deep! "But we never", "but we always", and "yeah, but" become the statements that signal such stagnant, "I'd-better-do-it" behavior.

It does not take a Rhodes scholar to figure out that as an agency or program grows in service to others, that one person cannot do all the things that need to be done. Founders of organizations frequently forget this point and continue to try to do everything, make all decisions, control all aspects of work, etc. Eventually of course, things fall apart, with the founder claiming too little time and not enough appreciation. Unfortunately ministers frequently fall into the same pattern.

The root of the problem is one of reluctance to relinquish control, thus preventing real delegation to others of major, whole responsibilities. This type of disabling manager (a manager has only two choices — to enable or disable others!) is usually very clever and frequently seems to delegate — but actually only gives out bits and pieces of work, witholds authority or takes back what has been "delegated" when the worker doesn't do something exactly as they would have.

Poor job descriptions, or lack of any at all, are another valley in the landscape of poor management.

Nothing is more critical to ultimate success than having the people involved know what they are to do, when, where, and in relationship to all "others" doing related work.

You'd be amazed at how many programs in the helping professions still do not have clear, concise, make-sense descriptions of what each person is to do.

I had one of the top five charities in America send me their "job descriptions" for their top field positions, asking me to critique them. It was probably fortunate the person who sent them wasn't present when I received and read them. They might have had a clue from my gagging that there was something wrong.

One description, for a state director, went on for seven pages. It was either written by a highly intelligent expert in Sanscrit or an illiterate chimpanzee as its rhetoric was indecipherable. After reading it I had no idea of what the job entailed, how long they would do it, who they reported to, what support they would get, how they would be evaluated, or what their duties were (minor details).

As I looked through each job description the charity had sent me, I began to laugh hysterically and pull on my lower lip. Since this behavior closely resembled what the charity had described as that of their many employees and volunteers, I felt I was qualified to critique their job descriptions!

Too frequently the lack of clear descriptions of what each person is to do and their inter-relationships is the real cause of problems rather than the handy excuse of "too little time." Can you even guess at how much time is wasted as everyone runs around wondering what the heck they are supposed to be doing as they try to look busy?

The third culprit in poor management is the lack of understanding throughout the ranks of what the overall or individual project goals are for the group.

This lack of clarity of knowing where we're going can waste more time than the annual "Procrastinator-of-the-Year" award winner.

Time is given to frustration, false starts, wasted effort, and discussions of discontent in an organization aimed everywhere and nowhere.

Expectations of workers who go off "in the wrong direction" become dashed, and the seeds for a poor organizational climate are sown when people feel their time has been wasted in pursuit of a nondescript goal.

"Time" becomes a handy scapegoat to cover up the crimes of this lack of direction, which usually is the sign of poor leadership.

Poor delegation, job designs, and vision all can be the root problems hidden beneath the excuse of not enough time. Be careful not to be fooled by such a smoke screen. Time is not an enemy but an opportunity. Used wisely it feeds success, used poorly it feeds failure.

3. *Lack of Skills and Time* — I once had to deal with a conference planner for an event I was keynoting that kept complaining about her lack of time to properly put the conference together. She expected 100-200 people she said, "If I can just find the time to plan it."

Being a rather logical person, I had to question her statements since she started one year in advance and began her first contact to me with this complaint.

As the event drew closer, her wails became louder and more specific. I wished several times that I could come up with a reason to cancel out of what I knew would be a disaster. Since this was unethical, I hung in there, booking my plane ticket at the last moment in hopes that she'd cancel her fiasco.

She didn't. I went. Eleven people came. Gag.

After the disaster I had to listen to her during the trip back to the airport, as she blamed the problems on "too little time." When I pointed out she'd begun the year before she told me she needed 18 months.

At first I tried to help her examine each aspect — planning, marketing, scheduling, etc. to see what she might learn for the future. Soon however, I dropped this approach and resorted to scenery-watching and an occasional "hu-huh" to counterpoint her babbling excuses.

I recognized the real problem — she simply lacked the skills to plan a conference. I knew she was successful at managing a volunteer group locally. She was a whiz at a computer and won prizes for her counted cross stitch, but conference planning was not a gift!

One problem helping professionals seem to take on, is a belief that they can be all things to all people.

The excuse we often use for stumbling in our efforts is time constraints. We frequently make this excuse a self-fulfilling prophecy by having to expend so much time spinning our wheels, trying to figure out what we're supposed to do, berating ourselves for not being "good enough" and having to redo what we've done incorrectly the first, second or third time around.

The question of "If you can't find the time to do it right, how you find the time to do it over?" takes on new meaning for the person who lacks skills for an assignment.

As managers of others, we are called upon to place "right people in right jobs" — making sure that the assigned worker has the necessary skills or learning ability to accomplish the goal successfully.

To be a better steward of our own time and therefore our own self, we need to also assess those assignments we might accept personally in line with our individual skill levels.

Time is not an enemy. Frequently it is an excuse for other behavior that leads to failure or shortfalls. Time is not found or made, it simply is.

What we do with our time is what's important, for it is all we have available to us. It is the framework for our accomplishments and experiences.

How we utilize it determines if it is friend or foe to our wholistic health and well-being.

If we see it as a friend, it will support and uphold us. If we see it as foe it will frustrate and restrain us.

The choice is ours.

CONCLUSION ...

The quiet killers that present the greatest threat to our taking care of ourselves are a rather crafty, insidious lot.

Grief, burnout, stress, guilt, confusion between worth and work, keeping score, and time can erode our physical, emotional, mental, spiritual, and relational health from within with disasterous results.

But our best defense against them is a constant awareness of our internal messages — a continual assessment of what's really going on inside of ourselves.

82

When we are aware of these internal enemies we can put them in their proper place or perspective, usually by balancing reality with expectations, and be free of their negative messages.

The key defense against these quiet killers is, I believe, a healthy attitude of self-worth with a liberal dose of self-forgiveness thrown in.

When we believe in ourselves, our value as a person, our best efforts and our systems, we are equipped to handle all of these potential killers handily.

CHAPTER II
END NOTES

1. Westburg, Granger. *Good Grief.* Fortress Press, PA. 1962.

2. University of Colorado. Volunteer Management Workshop. Dept. of Conferences. Boulder, CO 80306.

3. Maslach, Christina. *Burnout. The Cost of Caring.* Prentice-Hall. 1982.

4. Maslach, Christina. Burnout Inventory. *Burnout — The Cost of Caring,* Prentice-Hall. Englewood Cliffs, NJ. 1982.

5. Ibid. p. 58.

6. Jaffee, Dennis and Scott, Cynthia. *From Burnout to Balance,* McGraw-Hill, NY. 1984, p.4.

7. Ibid. pp. 5 & 6.

8. Ibid. p. 8.

9. Jud, Robert. *Straight Talk About Stress,* Executive Female. Mar/Apr 1985.

10. Kushner, Harold. *When Bad Things Happen to Good People.* Avon Books, NY. 1981.

11. Sergeant, Alice. *Androgynous Manager.* AMA Com. 1981.

12. Schramm, Mary. *Gifts of Grace.*

13. Larkin, Alan. *How to Get Control of Your Time and Your Life.* Video Tape.

14. Wilson, Marlene. *Survival Skills for Managers,* Volunteer Management Associates, Boulder, CO 1981.

CHAPTER III

DIMENSIONS

THE SUPER-DIMENSION ...

For many years I have heard about our four primary dimensions ... physical, mental, emotional, and spiritual. Recently however, the more I thought about these four, the more I became convinced that there was a fifth dimension that really was most critical of all as we look at the question of how to take care of ourselves.

That dimension is "relational" and intertwines itself with all the other four.

In discussing wellness and how caregivers can attain and maintain balanced health for themselves, I do not mean that everyone of us must be physical amazons, mental geniuses, emotional stalwarts, or spiritual giants 100% of the time. That's irrational and impossible.

While I was recuperating from my surgery for the colostomy I was still what I considered to be "well" in <u>relation</u> to my physical being, though I was far from well at first and much removed from any such definition as "physical amazon." The key factor was that I was at "peace" with my physical essence and not angry at my limitations.

How we relate to our four primary dimensions is of greater importance than being totally capable. Therefore, a quadriplegic I know of is in harmony with her physical dimension because she has come to peace with that aspect of her life and could therefore be described as healthy.

Jo Coudert in her book Advice from a Failure states: "peaceful coexistance with all parts of the self turns one loose to go about the business of living with equanimity."[1]

When I was trying to adjust to my colostomy and experiencing flashbacks to near-death incidents in the hospital, I would have been described as emotionally raw by psychologists, yet I realized that those experiences were a part of my recovery. My relationship to my emotional dimension was, therefore, healthy even during the time of a great fragility of my emotions.

One of the most frustrating times for me was the first few weeks after the colostomy when, due to effects of the peritonitis and subsequent medications and pain killers, I had difficulty thinking clearly or making decisions.

Since I pride myself on my mental agility, this became a real source of concern and self-directed anger until I recalled Elaine Yarbrough's suggestion to enter into a "neutral zone" when a major change occurs, to give yourself time to adjust.

In recalling her words and following her advice, I really turned my mental flame down to "low," and in so doing, found a healthy relationship to it.

Like all the other three primary dimensions, we have highs and lows, even "ons" and "offs" to our spiritual dimension. There are times we feel very close to and guided by our spiritual God. At other times we wonder about the existence of God and His distance from us.

Again the key to feeling healthy and whole is our relationship with our spiritual side. Is the relationship one of harmony or discord, of reality or fantasy, of peace or war?

We must be careful here not to judge others with our own measuring stick. Some of the people I've known who seem to me to exemplify the most beautiful relationship with God have been at odds with the organized church (including some ministers I know!) and several people who carried a Bible around, spent more time in church than anywhere else and spouted scripture in every conversation were actually most in disharmony with their spiritual dimension.

Also, we must be careful not to downgrade or discount the spirituality of people from religions or philosophies different from our own.

I become very uncomfortable when I hear someone insisting that people who do not march to the exact same spiritual drummer as themselves are "lost" and damned for their beliefs. Sounds a little too much like playing God to me!

The point is, of course, not how strong or good you are physically, mentally, emotionally, or spiritually, but what relationship you have with each dimension . . . how you feel about any of these facets as they dynamically change through life's journey.

Are you at peace with what and who you are? Are you in harmony with yourself? Do you accept who you are, celebrating your strengths and forgiving your weaknesses?

Do you see gaps in any dimension that challenge you to work toward greater harmony and therefore wellness?

Have you attained the wisdom to know the difference between what you can change and what you can't, working on the former and letting go of the latter?

I cannot change the physical limitations of my life. The illness, surgery, colostomy, etc. will always be a part of my reality as Sue Vineyard. Limitations on my stamina and strength as they exist today are the facts of my life and must be dealt with.

My relationship to my physical dimension is the critical factor in my wellness. My acceptance, my adjustment, my adaptation, my peace of mind.

Having found a good and healthy relationship with my physical limitations brings me to a health-filled and whole existence.

I may function differently than the average person; I may also depend on the plastics industry for a full life; I may even have to endure embarrassing "accidents," but I feel good about myself and can say with a bright twinkle, "Have bag, will travel."

PHYSICAL HEALTH . . .

Through the years I have tried to play a game with myself regarding my physical dimension. The name of the game might be entitled "Let's Pretend" and refers to a norm I developed to pretend I was fine physically.

My early childhood physical dimension ran into its first roadblock when, at age 5, I contracted Typhoid Fever by drinking contaminated water while visiting my grandparents in Joliet, Illinois. In hindsight, doctors now tell me that is where I first developed weaknesses in my colon and started down the road that eventually led to a hospital emergency room in 1986.

Later childhood brought on several bouts with Rheumatic Fever that even continued into adulthood. Through all this, fatigue and "stomach problems" became so familiar that I took them to be normal, and simply went on about the business of living.

As I have tried to explain to several doctors who questioned my acceptance of chronic and constant discomfort in the digestive tract, I didn't realize that the way I was feeling physically was not the way everyone felt.

As physical beings, we have only ourselves to use as guides as to what "normal" is. Certainly, when acute pain or discomfort come about, we know something is amiss, but when all you can ever recall is eating followed by discomfort and several doctors (when you do question it) chalk it up to "nerves," you simply grit your teeth and think it's part of life.

In assessing our physical being, I feel it is important to understand what is normal and what is not. In looking back I can now identify several doctors that I should have pressed harder in having them investigate my problems, or have changed to medical personnel who listened to me wholistically. Had I been more forceful or more secure about myself, therefore rejecting the years of being told I was imagining my pain, I probably would have prevented the ruptured colon and years of discomfort through diverticulitis.

Even when the diverticulitis was diagnosed, the diet and medication first prescribed were, I found out later, exactly opposite and incorrect for my condition.

I once heard a medical doctor talking on television about medications and urging that when you get a new one prescribed, the sensible thing to do is go to the library and look it up so that you know what it is supposed to do, its side effects, and what ailments it is prescribed for. At the time I thought that that sounded rather extreme, but now I think it may sound rather practical. A check on the medication prescribed several years ago would have told me it was for colitis not diverticulitis. A check years ago on the Valium prescribed would have told me it was not a muscle relaxant as I was told but an anti-depressant. This would have saved me three days of confused thinking and dullness before I threw the pills in the garbage! (And would have diagnosed a gall-bladder attack much earlier.)

The reason I share all this is that I now believe it is not enough to simply tell people to listen to their bodies. We must also know what is truly normal and healthful from a physical sense and not be lured into thinking that a rather abnormal, yet life-long, pattern is healthy. I had this brought home to me recently by a friend calling to say she had just read an article on ringing in the ears (Tinitus) and was shocked to find that your ears aren't supposed to do that! All her life she heard a high pitched ring and thought that was the way everyone heard! In other words, what she considered normal was actually abnormal, so her evaluation of her physical wellness was tainted.

After having cautioned you thoroughly about knowing what normal and healthy really are, let me share how important I feel it is to listen to your body.

I did myself and therefore those who care about me, the greatest of disservices by ignoring my own body signals through the years. My adopted attitude of being a "good soldier" with a stiff upper lip during all the times I was feeling rotten was, I believe, an equal villain to stress in bringing me to death's door.

By ignoring physical symptoms for years, and even almost self-hypnotizing so that pain stayed compartmentalized away from my conscious mind, I erroded my body, my health, and my welfare with almost disastrous results.

In addition to this, I also was rather haphazard about caring for my physical being. Exercise was something I thought you did when you had a free moment (and I almost never had those!) or was left to the size 5, Jane Fonda types of the world.

As I watched runners jog by my house I discounted that option by looking at the pained expressions on their faces. "That doesn't look like much fun!" I thought as I chalked it off my list.

When my husband began to walk each night in rehabilitation after a heart attack, I checked that off the list with the excuse that I couldn't keep up with his long-legged stride. When it was suggested I find a female walking partner and I asked a neighbor, I now admit to feeling relieved when she couldn't work it into her schedule ("Well, I tried").

I became very creative in excuse-giving for not exercising physically and went blithly on with a pattern of high physical activity on the road and little at home as a counterpoint. I was asking my body to perform like an athlete for a few days a week then become a blob on off days.

The only time I walked was when I felt emotionally or mentally strained and therefore felt the need to "walk it off" . . . again, only when I had time.

This pattern, coupled with erratic eating habits of no appetite on the road and over eating at home with a high sugar content (I confess to being a chocoholic!) were playing havoc with my body, which through personal and family health history, was already programmed for problems.

In looking at your physical being in addition to norms and listening to your body, I urge you to pay careful attention to your family history. Only recently have I realized that that history in my life could have helped me take precautions in my youth or early adulthood, which again, might have prevented or curtailed the physical toll of the present days.

In my background I have a paternal Grandfather who died of rectal cancer, a maternal Grandfather and uncle who had most of their stomachs removed due to ulcers, a mother with ulcers, a father with several bouts of colon cancer, and a sister with colitus. Add to this patterns of breast cancer, strokes, arthritis, Parkinson's Disease and irregular heart rhythms and you can see a family health history that can spell concern.

In assessing your own physical well being, not only of today, but of the future, it is critical therefore, to look at it from various angles ... that of normal, healthy patterns which medical personnel can share with you; that of body signals, both subtle and overt, and your own and family health history.

To assess what you might like to change about your physical dimension, I urge you to look at the options that surround you and discuss them with a competent physican or health professional. In our area, we have several wholistic health facilities and an even larger number of physicians who believe in wholistic health medicine who can help you map out a plan of attack that is suited to you personally and does not put you in further danger from inappropriate action.

In such a plan all aspects of your physical well being need to be addressed: diet, exercise, medications, relaxation techniques, health patterns, energy levels, restrictions, etc. etc. Be careful not to try to simply copy another person's pattern because they are the physical specimen you would like to be. Don't become fanatical about your plan, allow yourself latitude, creativity, and most of all, flexibility. (I don't want you physically perfect but insane because you didn't lift weights for 20 minutes this morning!)

When all else fails, use common sense as you deal with your physical dimension, remembering that your own relationship to your physical side is as important as a slim waist and bulging biceps. How you feel about yourself in this dimension is a critical factor in your wholistic health, therefore explaining how the quadriplegic I know can feel good about her physical dimension even though she can move only her head.

Caregivers, who must care so totally for their clients, patients, volunteers, staff, students, etc. need to look carefully at their own physical being, assessing its wellness and not neglecting signs of fatigue, illness, or distress in their determination to serve others. Putting yourself aside to help ohers, is, in the long run, the greatest disservice you can do those you seek to help. If you don't take care of yourself, how can you take care of them?

There are many books which can help you achieve patterns of physical wellness. One such book is Super Immunity[2] by Paul Pearsall which not only examines our own body defenses against disease but speaks at length to the importance of finding medical personnel who will work in a team approach with you to personal wellness. The book offers many concrete suggestions for readers to attain physical health, respond positively to life, and to establish a positive and effective attitude.

OUR MENTAL HEALTH . . .

When I speak of mental health in this section I am focusing on the intellectual dimension of our being and its health. Elsewhere I refer to matters regarding our emotional mental health, and I think it is important to distinguish between the two.

As I have stated before, my mental agility became a great concern to me while I was still in the hospital in July as I was trying to think through a fog created by pain, medications, and infection. I can recall "testing" myself by trying to recall points I frequently use in training . . . imagine the surprise on the medical personnel's face had they been able to read my mind and discover I was reciting the list of the ten Megatrends, McClelland's motivational classifications or the five functions and ten components of the management process while being tended to!

Because it was difficult to speak due to weakness and tubes, I wasn't very good at conversation and writing letters was impossible, so I had to be content with trying to recall complex thoughts and rehearse them in my mind.

At first I probably would have gotten a C- as a grade, but as time went on my marks improved, and I began to believe that they really had only removed part of my colon and not part of my brain!

I would hope that you would not have such a catastrophic reason to "check out" your mental dimension, but I do urge that in looking at your wholistic health, you examine your intellectual dimension and attend to its needs.

One of the great blessings in my life, as I refer to several times in this book, is my relationship with three soulmates in my support system: Marlene Wilson, Arlene Schindler, and Elaine Yarbrough.

These wonderful all-accepting people have provided me with an acid test and exercise of my mental dimensions as we banter, discuss, explore, and stretch in our conversations. In looking back to one particular weekend we spent in the Colorado mountains, I recall our discussions ranging from shoes to the American touch cultures, from the benefits of massage to the cosmos. Between such diverse topics came lists of books we referred to one another for reading, a lot of laughter, and some deep counseling on subjects of concern to one or the other of us.

I came away from that weekend more refreshed than ever before. Much of that refreshment came from the fact that all of my dimensions . . . physical (we took long walks in the mountains, soaked in hot tubs, and ate very healthy food); relational (what joy to be with such loving friends!); emotional (it was a time of such trust that any emotion could be expressed); spiritual (we probably talked most about God and our relationship with Him) and mental (much like a mental calesthentics class!) . . . were being tended to. Also, however, I realize then I had <u>never</u> been so mentally challenged and stimulated as when I was with these three remarkable people.

I believe that after that weekend I was more convinced than ever of the need to stay mentally healthy, working to continue to be a life long learner, trying new ideas, exploring new thoughts, stretching in all directions.

It also helped me realize a trait I have in my character which is that doing the same thing for too long a time becomes mentally boring to me and is no longer a challenge. This realization and the acceptance of it as neither good nor bad, helped me to identify my need to infuse my training with new thoughts and readings and to explore new subject matter that would challenge me as I worked on new presentations.

In assessing and tending to my wholistic health today, this realization has prompted me into several new ventures and avenues. I have agreed to do some counseling with ostomy patients locally with my new friend and ostomy specialist, Jean Parker; I am making five video tapes on volunteer management, marketing, and trends for release; I am developing an entirely new training session on care for the caregiver plus writing this book. All of these avenues are demanding a great deal of new learning and stretching as I try to bring the best of myself to each project.

Sadly, I am acquainted with a woman, who though extremely bright, has shut down her mental dimension and refuses to explore new thoughts and learnings. Through this pattern she has become convinced that she is no longer bright and even wonders if she is suffering some brain damage or illness to account for what she labels dullness. In observing and talking to her, it is clear that she has voluntarily shut down her intellectual dimension in grief over an imposed circumstances in her life (poor health of a spouse). She has erected a wall around her with a major barrier being her refusal of almost all intellectual stimulation and even the use of the mental skills she aready has.

The fallout of this choice, to shut down intellectually, is that emotionally she is very depressed, socially she has isolated herself, physically she is demonstrating classic symptoms of stress-related illnesses, and spiritually she is empty. I fear for the lady's very existance as her wholstic health crumbles around her.

We cannot ignore any aspect of our whole self, as a deficiency in any one of the five dimensions can and will effect the others negatively. Our mental or intellectual facet is of key importance to a balanced wellness and benefits not only ourselves but others close by and the world in general as we remain contributing, alert, and creative partners in the body of learning we call life.

Examine the opportunities you have in your life to stretch intellectually, to grow mentally, and to discover the joys found in new thoughts, perspectives, and ideas. How much time do you make in your life for refreshing mentally? Who can you be with that can stimulate you intellectually?

I have a dear friend who spends one morning each week pouring over the New York Times, cutting out stories on things she has little knowledge of so that she can explore them more fully, identifying those articles she feels can be of benefit in her own work or others she knows (I frequently get items from her that pertain to my work), or simply things she feels are interesting. She uses it as a mental exercise and an "expansion tool" in her determinaion to continue to grow and learn.

Obviously, my friend with her New York Times exercise is a curious person. I find that curiosity is a trait I admire deeply in others and myself. I am reminded of one of the greatest joys I found in young motherhood, the curiosity of both of my sons as they discovered the world. How I loved to show something new to them and see how they responded to and interpreted it.

I especially recall a Sunday after church school when my oldest son Bill came out of his classroom so excited he could barely talk. At five he had experienced a whole new phenomenon, and he could not wait until he shared it with me, sure of course that no one had ever noted it before!

He grabbed me by the hand and pulled me in the class to view two new friends that he had obviously ordered to "stand here til my

Mom sees you." When I looked at them I was startled myself to see two of the most identical twins I had ever laid eyes on, but even more delighted with Bill's description of them which explained the phenomenon perfectly . . .

"Look Mom," he squeeled, "God made two same-guys!"

From that day forth, the Olson twins were known in our house as those "Same-guys," and the word has stuck to this day when we are referring to identical twins!

Bill was expressing both his curiosity and his delight at a new discovery. In this instance and in thousands more our sons looked at life as a wonderful mystery waiting to be solved and holding treasures to be discovered.

If we as adults can recapture some of our youthful curiosity we will, as a result, keep our intellectual dimension hale, hearty, and healthful. Not all of us can be mental genuises, but we can stretch toward our own horizons as we remain life long learners, and in so doing, find mental health and growth.

EMOTIONAL HEALTH
WHAT YOU SEE IS WHAT YOU GET . . .

I have a dear friend whose mother is going through a horrendously trying time. The mother, at 68, is faced with a husband who is suffering from Alzheimer's and Parkenson's Diseases. Through 50 years of marriage her husband made all the decisions, took care of all financial and business matters, and basically shouldered all responsibilities for their life, future, etc.

You can imagine how overwhelmed she is now as she watches her husband withdraw further each day from reality and any ability to continue to be responsible for their lives.

Tragically for all involved her response has been to decide that she is now and always has been worthless, dull, and incapable. With this frame of reference she has sunk into dangerous depression. She has become non-functioning, sad, and with suicidal thoughts and anticipation of disaster at every turn.

The painful anticipations become self-fulfilling prophecies in a vicious cycle of defining failure as success ("See, I told you I couldn't do it!).

I have another friend, who is now in her 80's who has suffered many pains during her lifetime, including her husband's illness and death, who is still one of my town's "movers and shakers" as she leads community efforts.

To me these two women seem to be the opposite ends of the pendulum in regard to their emotional response to life.

As I try to understand what circumstances brought each to their present place in life (and to learn from what each can teach us) I find two major differences in their background:

1. By a series of circumstances my friend's mother frames all of life negatively; the other frames everything positively. One has the attitude of "I can't" the other, "I can try." Both are right.

2. My friend's mother led a life "free" of major responsibilities as her husband, out of love and duty, "took care" of her. She was therefore not given the chance to develop a sense of self-worth; a sense of "Wow! I can do that" many of us are familiar with when we stretch and meet a new challenge. My 80 year old friend, on the other hand, had a marriage partnership that encouraged her own growth and independence, exploration, and the opportunity to enrich her self-confidence.

The real lessons to be learned from these stories are again two-fold, especially for the helping professionals and caregivers of the world:

1. Our emotional framework for looking at life is critical to how we live that life. This framework is made up of our own self perception.

2. Making people dependent on us can create the greatest of handicaps.

I was delighted to find a book by John Powell, Associate Professor at Loyola University, entitled Fully Human, Fully Alive[3] that talks in depth about the first lesson.

In the introduction to the book, Powell states:

> "It now seems obvious to me that our emotional reactions are not permanent parts of our makeup, the way we were in the beginning, are now and ever shall be. Rather than grow out of the way we see ourselves, other people, life, the world and God. Our perceptions become the habitual frame of reference within which we act and react. Our ideas and attitudes generate our emotional responses. Persistently negative emotions are an indication that there is a distortion or delusion in our thinking, an astigmatism in our vision."

He also states, "But it is always this vision, (self-perception) however modified, that controls the quality of and participation in human life.[4]

As caregivers, I believe it is vital to continually check our self-perception, frame of reference and vision to see if it is real or distorted, positive or negative as the effect of this self-perception also frames our emotional health.

As we examine our emotional health we need to identify any undesirable patterns that exist — depression, anger, rage, sarcasm, skepticism, negativism, etc. and explore the probability that they are a result of the framework through which we look at life — our own self-perception.

Frequently as I talk with people who are sharing a frustration or a problem, I hear a self-perception that is causing a stumbling block.

"I'm not very creative" says the person who can't think of a new way to tackle a problem; "I'm not very well educated" (AKA: "I'm not too smart") says the person trying without success to learn how to use a computer; "I can't speak in front of a group" says the person unable to carry their story to the public; "I'm too old to learn something new" says the manager threatened by new ideas.

In each case, the person speaking has predetermined their success or failure by an emotional self-perception that frames all of their activities, decisions, choices, patterns, etc.

At times when you are checking your emotional help and self-perception, it is most helpful to have a significant other to help you in your assessment.

First of all, this "other" can offer you the emotional support and unconditional love that gives you the confidence to explore yourself deeply. It can also provide a definition of "you" as good and worthwhile from the perception of someone you value and who loves you.

It is necessary that this other person is a totally trusted confidant, to whom you feel free to say anything. You need to be free from inhibitions that might stop you from saying whatever you really feel, without becoming overwhelmed with embarrassment or reserve.

If during this self-inventory, you uncover negative visions of yourself, check them out with your significant other. Frequently you will find that even though you feel uncreative, your friend may see something quite the opposite and give you concrete examples of this perspective.

A second benefit may come from identifying those things you labeled as negative which are actual traits you possess but are not truly negative. I can recall identifying in myself my lack of skill in the art of "small talk." By discussing this with a soulmate, and admitting I felt this was a weakness of mine, I discovered two things: 1) I really wasn't so bad at it as I was repulsed by it — I don't like or value small talk! and 2) Not liking small talk is not a bad trait.

I modified an exercise a friend shares in her training sessions, whereby you list things you feel you don't do well and try to find value in this "non-ability."

As I looked for value in not liking small talk or doing it well, I listed:

1) Saves a lot of my time (and others)
2) Allows me to rest as I side-step social invitations I know will be full of it!
3) Conserves my energy for more valuable conversation and actions.

After examining the negative framework that had surrounded my self-perception as a flawed small-talker, I changed my vision to value this here-to-fore perceived weakness and turn it into a strength.

Too frequently I find helping professionals who have become their own worst enemy as they frame their self-perception with "I can't," "I'll never," "I'm not," or "I'm too old, handicapped, undereducated, impoverished, untalented, worthless, incapable, etc. to . . . "

In each instance, they have predetermined their success (or lack of it) by limiting their own vision.

I've also benefited from the opposite side of this coin by people perceiving me as an "expert," therefore finding success by what they feel I told them to do from my "expert" background. (Actually, in consulting with others, I find people already have the solutions to their concerns but need someone else to affirm their conclusions.) When they predetermine or pre-call the successful outcome of their actions, they will usually attain that success. It has nothing to do with my expert suggestion, but their vision of a positive outcome; their belief that it will come to a fruitful conclusion!

The moral of all this is: "What you see is what you get!".

If you see life, complete with its challenges, curves, surprises, and upheavals through a framework of emotional self-confidence and positive success, your results will fall into that mold.

If you see life through a framework of self-doubt, depression, "I can't," and negativism, the results will verify that vision too.

Emotional health is determined to a great extent by the way you "see" life. What is your framework for living? Your self-perception? Your vision?

If you think you can or you think you can't . . . you're correct!

WHEN HELPERS HELP TOO MUCH . . .

In looking again at the differences between my friend's mother and my 80 year old acquaintance, the second thing that strikes me is how other people's helping affects us.

In one instance, a husband lovingly carried almost all of the responsibility for decisions, problems, and life. This kept his wife from learning coping and practical skills she now needs to deal with his illness.

His intentions cannot be questioned — he was brought up in an era where the male head of the household took "care" of his wife and family. His purpose was to help and in fact, by many definitions, he probably seemed like a real gem as he shouldered all but the basic household functioning himself.

In looking at the result of his "helping" we now see a very angry woman unable to cope and emotionally crippled. Her anger is directed at her husband (which starts a guilt cycle!), and so the helper now becomes the target of recrimination — or to put it more precisely — the helper becomes the persecutor and eventually the victim.

As in all of life, there are shades and degrees of this cycle, but the eventual outcome of "victim" usually comes about when helping becomes excessive or inappropriate.

As caregivers we need to constantly assess our roles as helper. When does "helper" become "rescuer"? When does helping really hurt? What are the long term effects (on both you and those you try to help) of your helping?

A deeper level of exploration must take place around the issue of why you are helping.

I have met many people who help others out of their own need more than the "others." Rarely do I find a person who understands or will admit this.

I realize now that I had confused who the real benefactor was as I tried to help everyone with the problems they brought to my doorstep. I kept telling myself "they" needed me, when in fact, I needed to be needed and seen as a helping, all-wise person.

What a web I entangled around me when I began to resent demands on my time beyond the training I'd been hired to do and subsequently felt guilt about such feelings.

At first, I masked my feelings of resentment by telling myself "They just don't understand what they're asking." This escalated to "They really don't appreciate what I'm giving them" and finally to "I can't stand anyone else taking hunks of me! What do they think I am?"

When I'd gotten to this final, rather angry stage, I began to clock and calendar watch as I tried to simply survive my travel schedule. I kept scheduling "times off" between trips to try to break the grip of exhaustion and emptiness I felt.

I ignored several soulmates expressions of concern and caution as they saw what I was doing to myself but somehow couldn't stop.

As I continued to book myself too tightly, stay up late listening to others, and throw myself into a dramatic frenzy on stage, I really was trying to feed my own needs to be seen as a "helper" rather than anyone else's needs to be helped.

What an ah-ha! I had one night after a particularly grueling day of training and listening to problems when a dear friend, Arlene Schindler, challenged me about whether any extra counseling was done because the counselees needed it or I did!

What opened up in my mind's eye by addressing that question was a whole new awareness of my needing to live up to my own self image of helper, listener, compassionate counselor, etc. Obviously the only way to do so was to send out signals constantly of "Come to me — I'll help."

Somehow I'd managed to turn the helper-persecutor-victim cycle in on myself! With the ultimate victimization being a decline in my own physical health.

In regard to others, I can recall a classic case of a top executive in volunteerism deciding to mentor several other people in an attempt to help them increase their skills, advance rapidly, and become more effective.

Hours, days, and months were spent sharing, guiding and assisting her fledglings. Soon however, a "kink" developed in the executive's relationships with two of her mentees. A subtle change shifted as the executive went from helper to rescuer when problems arose.

Suggestions that were offered were labeled as demands and resented; guidance was branded as interference; concern as nosiness; example-setting as prima-donna-like behavior.

The executive was bewildered and hurt. Pain replaced pleasure as everyone tried to pretend everything was fine. (Helping professionals rarely acknowledge conflict — that's not "nice.)

It was a classic case of helper becoming persecutor and finally victim. Two of the people being mentored became angry and defiant of their mentor. A classic power struggle resulted aimed at control of the business. One of the two problem persons even wanted the executive to name a successor if she died! (And when she wouldn't, became more punitive in her interaction with the executive!)

It finally came down to the only possible resolution being the dissolution of the relationship — all because in good intention, one person who wanted to "help" slipped over into the dangerous position of becoming a "rescuer" and was eventually persecuted, becoming a victim.

Another subtle variance of this helping-persecuting-victim cycle centered around a marvelous and much lauded church training program for the laity. As its success grew the hierarchy of the church in question became very threatened by the way the program was helping congregations toward more meaningful ministry of lay people as they tapped into awareness and utilization of individual and collective gifts.

Demands on the leaders of the program were increased to a ridiculously impossible level. Funding was cut. Design changes were demanded. Debates centered on wordings began, and every subtle way was devised to discourage the leaders of the program. Persecution ran rampant!

Finally the program was cancelled as "non priority" with vague promises to resurrect it in a new form (AKA: watered down and minus the originating leadership). The program and its leadership, became the victim.

Its only crime was it helped too <u>much</u> — it was too successful and was stirring up questions of "Who's in charge? Who's in control?"

All of us need to look at the whole question of helping, examining the real motivations behind helping; when helping becomes rescuing; how too much helping can cripple others; and when we need to break any cycle that can lead us from helper to persecuted to victim.

We are in the business of helping, yet like anything, it can be done to excess, masked in good intentions and hidden agendas. We need to find healthy, balanced ways to offer our help in a manner that truly accomplishes our goal of enabling rather than disabling.

In so doing we take a giant stride toward balanced and effective emotional health . . . of ourselves and others!"

ASSESSING SPIRITUAL HEALTH . . .

Different people will define the word "spiritual" in various ways.

Many will associate it with their own religion and a specific church. Doctrine as well as tradition is a great factor in their spiritual life.

Others will take a broader view and define it as their wider relationship with God; their faith in a source of power far beyond any one church.

Still others will translate "spiritual" as their own "spirit" - their attitudes and feelings that surround the actions of their lives. Their focus is on the spiritual within them rather than without.

Obviously, these three different types will find different ways to assess spiritual strength and opportunities for growth.

The first will usually find refreshment from litergy and rituals, visiting their home church, speaking to their pastor, etc.

The second will often be renewed by a good Bible or religious study group, or talking with various people of great faith irregardless of their "brand" or designation. Nature can offer them great uplifting of the spirit as they are reminded of God's creatave power, and they often appreciate great wisdom as revealed through other, very different religions from theirs.

The third will usually seek people or actions that can lift their spirits. Again nature can offer this to them, as well as discussions of values with close friends, intellectual explorations of spiritual issues, the revelations that come through hearing a good seminar leader, the satisfaction of doing good works for others. They may or may not be "in tune" with a God-head figure beyond themselves.

Your list, therefore, of ways to strengthen your spiritual health will be a highly personal one. There are no right answers to such a listing — no "better" or "worse" paths to spiritual health.

The purpose is to focus on this facet of your life — to assess its present strength, to find ways to make it even stronger and to identify any aspects of this all important facet that need "shoring up."

I would first urge you to identify how important this part of your life is to you. You cannot deny its existence (though some will try) as we all have a spiritual side — whether or not we also define that as religious.

Our attitudes, moods, feelings, hope, faith, etc. are part of this spiritual side of us and often define how we "do" things, how much energy we feel we have to go about the business of life and certainly how we make choices for the present and the future.

Ask yourself:
Do I feel I have a spiritual side to me?
Is it a predominant factor in my life?
Am I hopeful for the future because or
   in spite of it?
Do I recognize attitude as a factor in my life?
Do I only associate spirituality with religion?
Do I feel I am the total power in my life or is
   there something beyond me?
Do I believe in God?
What is my relationship with God?

By looking at your answers, a pattern will probably emerge of your attention to the spiritual aspect of your life. Is it a conscious part of your daily life or a part of you you keep hidden away in the corners of your mind — never acknowledged, dealt with, or examined?

Another thing in your self-examination that needs to be considered is: Is your present spiritual awareness/life different from previous times in your life?

Are you more or less in tune with your spirituality now than at other times of your life? Does your spirituality have different characteristics today than before? Does your spiritual being seem like a friend, a foe or a stranger, and how does that differ from previous perceptions?

Obviously, you are looking at where you are in relation to this facet in your life. Only you can answer the questions posed. Only you can assess your satisfaction with this part of your life.

I urge you to not only acknowledge this part of your being, but the importance it has in a totally healthy "you." When careful attention is given to the spiritual facet of your being you will find greater balance for yourself and therefore greater wholistic health.

WHERE DO I NOW FEEL IN TOUCH WITH MY SPIRITUAL SIDE?

> at church
> in nature
> reading the Bible
> prayer
> prayer groups
> with others of like-thinking
> with clergy
> Bible studies
> with people I think
>   are very spiritual themselves
> during alone time
> on retreats
> during church rituals
> in discussions with others
> with my support group
> during activities I enjoy, such as:
> other _____
>
> _____
>
> _____

WHERE MIGHT I GO TO RENEW SPIRITUALLY?

    church
    Bible studies
    nature
    visits with family
    visits with friends/loved ones
    activity: _____
    seminars
    school classes
    talks with clergy
    talks with professional counselors
    silent times
    other: _____

    _____

    _____

IS ANYBODY UP THERE? . . .

Before I even put one word of this section down, I know it's going to make a lot of people angry.

Some will be angry because I don't say the expected, "usual" things about God and spiritual strength, others because I included such a chapter at all.

Even talking about spiritual subjects seems to lead to problems.

I can recall training in Florida for about 100 clergy and lay leaders on the topic of Volunteerism in the Church. The evaluations were glowing, and I received many comments of "right on!" and "I wish more people could hear you talk about this subject; We've sure been misusing the gifts volunteers offer us for a long time."

When I got home, I received two strongly stated letters. One was from a male clergyman who said he was disappointed that I did not refer to God in the traditional sense of the male figurehead, and therefore he questioned whether I was a true Christian.

The second was from a female lay leader in a church who blasted me (in very unlady-like words) because I had referred, during the eight hours of training, to God as "He" and that I was, therefore, a sexist, a "failed Christian" (whatever that means) and condemmed to eternal damnation. She went on to state that she planned to devote a great deal of her time to ruining my career as a trainer, which, she stated was what I deserved.

I was tempted to write them both back, sharing some thoughts on "Grace," but decided that such a response was fruitless on my part and would fall on deaf ears. Instead, I filed it away in my mind's eye, in a collection of examples of disturbing encounters with people who present themselves as part of the army of God.

My own spiritual journey has been a life-long one, complete with fits and starts, two steps forward, then one step backward. Fortunately, God is patient, and never gives up on me, knowing, I suppose, that I belong to Him and that I'm trying to follow His lead for my life.

Let me share that I have come to a relationship with God that is quite opposite any picture of an old man with a long white beard, sitting on a golden throne dictating every twitch of my nose.

I also reject the God of "Gottcha" that several people I know seem to worship . . . the God who sits around waiting for you to do something wrong so He can pounce on you with punishment and anguish.

The God I love is my friend. When I, through the free will He gave me, get myself into hot water, he steadies me as I work my way out of the mess. When I hurt, He is the first to cry and when I rejoice, He is the first to clap His hands in glee.

He has a great sense of humor, and we chuckle together often at what goes on around us. He has the greatest wisdom, which He shared through His son, Jesus, but which I seem to keep forgetting and have to be reminded of over and over.

He's the strongest of the strong, and carries me when I can't carry the burdens of life by myseslf. Unfortunately, I keep forgetting He'll do this for me if I just ask, and therefore I've tried to carry too many burdens all by myself, bending and even breaking at the task.

To remind myself of His support, I have a card in my wallet with the poem "Footprints in the Sand" which helps remind me of the constancy of His love:

> "One night I had a dream. I was walking along the beach with the Lord, and across the skies flashed scenes from my life. In each scene I noticed two sets of footprints in the sand. One was mine, and one was the Lord's. When the last scene of my life appeared before me, I looked back at the footprints in the sand, and, to my surprise, I noticed that many times along the path of my life there was only one set of footprints. And I noticed that it was at the lowest and saddest times in my life. I asked the Lord about it: "Lord, you said that once I decided to follow you, you would walk wih me all the way. But I notice that during the most troublesome times in my life there is only one set of footprints. I don't understand why you left my side when I needed you the most." The Lord said: "My precious child, I never left you during your time of trial. Where you see only one set of footprints, I was carrying you."

Throughout my life He's given me innumerable gifts: talent, skills, relationships, knowledge, love, community, etc. etc. I try not to take them for granted, but sometimes I get cocky and think they are of my own doing, at which time He proves His loving patience with me, until I remember to thank Him again for the gifts.

Through the last few years, I realized I was storing up a lot of unhealthy feelings of anger and frustration at the organized church. I kept tripping over people who, in the name of God, were going around pointing fingers at others, judging them as "good" or "bad." I even dealt closely with a few who began to pronounce all those who disagreed with their definition of God as disciples of Satan.

I also had to deal with church officials who seemed to worship at the altar of mediocrity and personal power. One high ranking official of a Protestant church told me that the main problem with churches was "the stupid laity." Another argued that the word "volunteer" could not be used in my training because the word "disciple" was the only acceptable word. Yet another, in a personal encounter, shared his belief that "strong" people such as myself, really didn't need support from a Pastor.

Some of the worst horror stories seem to come from the church in regards to being misused, burned out, and invalidated. Lay leaders tell me that when they finally got a good volunteer program going in the church a minister or group of other lay leaders made sure it was squashed. Pastors tell me of their efforts to help people share their gifts only to have a church council reprimand them for "straying outside of the work we called you to do."

I seemed to be accumulating a long list of examples of people going to the well to drink only to have to pay too heavy a price for the water or having someone block their way.

In my reflections since my surgery, and my continuing journey with God, I had to examine all my feelings in regard to the church and separate them from my feelings for God and spirituality in general. This was a first step in bringing my spiritual being to a healthier place.

I came to realize that in focusing on the horror stories, I was overlooking the good news of the gifts of devout, God-loving people from all faiths, Christian and non-Christian, who were part of my life. I also acknowledged that I had allowed my frustrations with people who were doing terrible things to others in the cloak of God-liness to obscure my view of God as He exists in myself and the people I encounter.

When I was National Director of a charity that served 22 countries and the USA, and which specialized in helping the children of poverty, I had an opportunity to travel to Guatemala and stay with an ancient Indian tribe there that our charity served. In the village, with its thatched roof huts, dirt paths and central open market, our charity had opened a clinic for dying and starving children. Besides critical care, we taught basic nutrition to mothers who would bring their children along during their "lessons."

One day while I and five others from our staff were visiting, we spent a morning in the clinic, working with the children who had come that day. One of the children, a tiny, emaciated little girl of five, sat amidst the other children who laughed and played around her, yet she had no expression on her face.

Her tiny hands laid motionless on her lap and no manner of coaxing by the clinic worker convinced her to participate in activities.

One of my Division Directors, Gary Thorud, of Atlanta, was attracted to this little waif and squatted down on the floor next to where she sat. He drew pictures for her, he patted her, he talked to her, he made silly faces for her, all with the same result . . . no response.

Finally, he just sat quietly next to her and held her hand. For a half hour or longer she sat stoically looking at his hand over hers. Finally she looked cautiously at him, then moved ever so slowly closer to him, resting her head on his shoulder and placing her other tiny hand over his. Her blank exprssion was replaced by a look of peace and contentment, and it was clear that this child, half starved already and looking toward a life of not more than 28 or 29 years of excruciatingly hard work and labor, was for the moment, feeling safe.

As I look back on that scene, with the child snuggled next to Gary contentedly, and Gary crying softly at his victory, I realize I was seeing God at work.

We tend to think that God comes roaring down from heaven to do monumental things, like parting seas, protecting children from plagues or moving mountains. Certainly, He can do such spectacular things, but more often He comes to us in much subtler, gentler ways. In that village of Guatemala, He was coming to comfort a small child of His through Gary, who chose to love this tiny frail little girl and to simply be with her for a few hours.

In our helping professions and through the caregivers of the world, we see God everyday, reaching out to people to help, to care, to offer comfort and support. We are constantly surrounded by examples of God through His sending of the Holy Spirit to each of us, doing His work. We are reminded that we all can choose to be ministers of God, and that that honor is not limited to a select few with backward collars or flowing robes.

As we deal with the problems of society we have a choice. We can see God around us, working through people in a loving, caring way, or we can blame God for the problems and add to our anguish by focusing on those people who bring harm and pain to others.

One choice will bring us greater peace and joy, thereby adding positively to our wholistic health by adding strength and support to our spiritual being.

The other choice will bring us pain, anguish and add to potential self-destruction as we focus on the negative and deny the gifts that surround us.

I once read that the Hebrew word for Satan was "hinderer." I can think of nothing that could hinder us more in our life's journey than to neglect our spiritual health.

The goal, I believe, is to find God within ourselves and others, to see Him behind the works of people who care, and to reject an imposed God who has been watered down to suit the needs of the human mind. God is a mystery. God is really neither male or female; not a noun but a verb . . . a word of action.

The word "He" is used because it is the word of the common people.

Jesus was neither a priest nor a theologian. He was a minister in the sense that he went to where people were and brought his message of love and harmony in the language that the people understood. He didn't need a huge organization behind him to get his message across. He didn't have to worry about operations manuals (other than the Old Testament) or salary scales or advertising slogans. He simply acted in the ways God showed him.

We have the same opportunities each day.

By examining our spiritual being, by making sure that it is refreshed, encouraged and uplifted, we can take a giant step toward caring for our-selves, and in the process, find new and positive ways to care for others.

WHY ME GOD?

There was a time in my life long ago, when my image of God more closely resembled the old, white-bearded man on the golden throne that I had picked up in some Sunday school class or other. Part of this image dictated that everything that happened was of God's doing.

By believing this, I thought that everything bad that happened was somehow in the master plan, along with everything good. The idea of free will simply had nothing to do with these concepts, and therefore the thought that some things simply happen due to circumstances or as consequences of choices didn't enter my mind.

107

When I came to believe that choice did indeed have much to do with events in a person's life, I had to reexamine my old idea that God sat in His heaven all day deciding every little thing, from the flat tire to the pimple, that happened to me.

What really challenged my thinking and concept of God was the tragedy that I saw around me, either through clients served by groups I worked with, or in my own personal life.

When a young friend of ours was electrocuted on the job at the tender age of 28, I found myself asking "Why God?" I realized that my questioning at that time was simply a continuation of the question, "Why me, God?" during several periods of my youth when I was seriously ill and denied the joy of being in school for months at a time, to share life with my friends.

Somehow, at the time of the tragedy of the death of our friend, I came to believe that a loving God would not strike down a young father and husband in the prime of his life, but that a set of circumstances of poor choices by a manufacturer and co-worker had brought about Ray's death. I felt that before any of the rest of us could weep, God cried for Ray and those he left behind.

As we encounter life's difficult times, either in our own lives or lives of those around us, I believe it is necessary for us to ascribe events to circumstances rather than a vengeful God waiting to strike us down for supposed infractions. (An excellent book on this subject is Harold Kushner's When Bad Things Happen To Good People.)

A Pastor I met recently told of a young Rabbi who was called to the home of a couple who had just been told that their only child, a daughter of 19, had died of an aneurysm while walking on her college campus. Because it was one of his first such calls since becoming a Rabbi, he wondered what he would possibly say to comfort the indescribable grief the parents must be suffering.

To his shock, when he went to their home, their first words were, "We didn't say the proper prayers on the last holy day."

In their statement, he realized their belief that God had struck down their daughter because of their infraction of a rule of the Synagogue, and he was horrified that their image of God was that of a vengeful, punishing Lord.

When people hold this image in their minds, attributing all tragic and sad events of their life to punishment for having dome something wrong, I believe they are carrying an unnecessary burden of guilt that is destructive and the exact opposite of what God wants for us.

A friend of mine I had not seen for some time happened to call at the time I was first hospitalized for diverticulitis, and in the conversation I related not only my hospitalization but some of the health problems of my immediate family, including a heart attack of my husbands, illnesses of my parents etc. Her response to me was worded carefully and cloaked in loving phrases, but basically said that God was obviously punishing me for having not followed his admonition to be subservient to my husband, as seen in the fact that I worked outside the home.

She went on to relate that it was just in time that she had seen the light and given up her career to submit totally to her husband, but that to remind her of her transgressions, God had caused her daughter to suffer in school.

Her message was clear. All the problems in my life were because I had been bad and needed (and deserved) punishing. The old "God of Gotcha!" again.

I cannot tell you how I felt when I hung up the phone from my conversation with her. I was angry, frustrated, sad, and disappointed. I had expected that this friend of many years and shared experiences, would be supportive of me . . . instead I felt as though someone had hit me wih a two-by-four! I did not believe what she was saying was in any way true, but I still had to deal with my disappointment in my friend and my sad awareness that a basic value difference existed between us that was probably irreconcilable.

Thinking like this person can lead to "Why Me God?" thinking, that is in reality, the anger stage of grief. By getting stuck at his point, harmful feelings of guilt, anger, even rage, can interfer with our healthy being.

When things get tough, I find that a better question than "Why Me?" is "What now, God?" By this I mean that I have accepted what is and must now move on to doing the best I can with the circumstances that exist. The moving on will not be easy, but it will be with God, either at my side, or if need be, carrying me. It implies a partnership that is open to new beginnings, healings and going on.

"What now, God?" looks to the future, altered as it will be from the way things were, hopeful and open to new avenues of living and serving. Possibly this statement is a way to reaffirm my belief that when one door closes another opens, leading us in a new direction that can be as exciting and challenging as any we have experienced in the past.

We must let go of any notion that there is any plot out to ruin our lives, to bring pain and suffering down on us or those we love, or that a scorecard is being kept that promises punishment for every little "failure" or "bad grade."

God has given us the gifts we need to live our lives. It is up to us to make the best possible choices to utilize those gifts and to lean on spiritual strengths to get us through those times when choices, consequences, or circumstances challenge us with painful events.

We don't look to heaven when something good happens in our life and ask, "Why me, God?" so why should we ask that when something bad happens?

Let's give up the notion of a punishing God and help others around us to do the same. I think God will clap His hands with glee when we do!

"Those who are the closest to grace are the most aware of the mysterious character of the gift they have been given."[5]

RELATIONSHIPS — THE GOLD OF LIVING . . .

In brushing so close to death and subsequently examining the whole phenomenon known as life, I was pleased to find that my top priority for many years was in its rightful place.

As a person who moved frequently when I was growing up due to my Dad's job transfers, I had come to believe at an early age that the most important thing on which we could spend our energy was that of relationships.

Relationships with others, self, and God.

I'm sure this realization shaped my adult life in human service and made me concentrate most of my energies in this direction.

Helping professionals and caregivers of all varieties seem to predominately concern themselves with relationships, working to make them effective, productive, and satisfying. Oddly enough, the work can sometimes become so overwhelming that personal relationships begin to take a back seat, tipping us "off balance" in our quest for wellness.

Keeping solid relationships in balance is, I believe, a major factor in caring for ourselves. I have already talked about our relationship with ourselves and God and here I would like to concentrate on relationships with others, to help you examine that critical aspect of your life — recognizing those relationships which build you up and those that tear you down, those that celebrate you and those that castigate you.

I believe such a self-analysis is critical to your wholistically, healthy "being" and affects enormously all the things that you do and are.

Soul Mates

We have innumerable acquaintances as we go through life. Some of them become friends, a lesser number become close friends.

If we are very fortunate we also connect with a few who become what I call "soul mates." Those people with whom we can be totally open, vulnerable and honest. Those people who celebrate our successes and never feel threatened or in competition with us. Those people who love us for what we are, where we are, when we are, and not what we do.

I have been blessed with several soul mates who are a great support and comfort to me and, because I value fun so much, are also great play mates.

For anyone who knows me well, the first soul mate that probably comes to mind in my life is Marlene Wilson, the field of Volunteerism's best known author and trainer.

Marlene and I have been blessed with also finding two others, Arlene Schindler (Vice President of Prison Fellowship) and Elaine Yarbrough (outstanding author, trainer and consultant) who make up a primary support group we laughingly call "Skrewe U." (Don't be offended — it's all in jest!)

All four of us train together at the University of Colorado's Volunteer Management Program which Marlene founded with Ivan Scheier in 1972 and still heads as faculty director. One evening, after a long day of training we went out for dinner (our first time as a foursome) and had one of those electric experiences that happens very infrequently.

We laughed, shared, enjoyed, and stimulated each other in every direction. We all sensed an instant bonding, a common need for such bonding and a determination to work to nurture the relationship.

From that dinner came our ficticious "Skrewe U." which meets twice annually, has its own motto, fight song, seal, and creed. Time has added our own T-shirts and dozens of pictures of the four of us sharing wonderful adventures in various settings.

During our time together, our discussions run the gamut from serious theological concerns to likes and dislikes in shoes; our activities from grappling with deep thoughts to singing in pig-latin in a hot tub!

All of us come away from these times together refreshed, renewed, supported, and invigorated. There is a freedom between us that is all-accepting, non-competitive, and challenging at the same time. There is time for sense and nonsense and the switches back and forth between the extremes would make a trapeze artist dizzy!

In short, we have become each other's soul mates and primary support group and the infrequency of our gatherings (we live in Illinois, Colorado, and Virginia) does not lessen the bonds between us.

While hospitalized I drew on the support of these three people, not just through their constant calls, notes, and gifts, but through the memories we share where each of us is so deeply valued and a part of one another.

111

In times of stress and trial I can think of no more important reservoir of strength and uplifting than such a support group or individual. I urge you to take time now to list those soul mates of your life who unconditionally accept and value you, who offer themselves to your emotional, spiritual, intellectual and physical needs in a selfless and productive way.

Beyond the three I have mentioned, I can count several others in the same category, and though they live as far away as Hawaii, D.C., Minnesota, and North Carolina, each offers me support, acceptance, and understanding.

Knowing of their love sustains me through all the difficult times of my life, and my hope is that in identifying your list of soul mates you will feel strengthened also.

I urge you to stop for a moment and actually list those close friends and soul mates in your life. List also the frequency of your interaction so that you are aware of the opportunities you have to refresh with them. Keep your list close at hand to remind you of your own personal support circle and tap into it frequently and with joy!

I share several quotes from Advice From A Failure by Jo Coudert here that express my own feelings on relationships:

> "You should make yourself gifts of friends who do not need, but thoroughly enjoy your company, and then keep those friends by not holding on to them."[6]

> "Most people ask of their friends that they understand them, but on balance I think I prefer a friend who understands himself."[7]

> "The valuable friends are those who make you expand, who make you feel more decent and wiser than you suspect yourself to be."[8]

> "The object of friendship is not to eradicate differences but to have a continuing dialogue despite them, without challenges and with enjoyment, for there must be two people in a friendship, not a sound and an echo, two distinct individuals each of whom accepts the uniqueness of the other and does not push for identity of out look or behavior."[9]

RELATIONSHIPS WITH OTHERS — ACCEPTING REALITY

One night in 1965 I attended a meeting of my local Junior Women's Club as a guest, to see if I might like to join their ranks.

112

I thoroughly enjoyed the evening, felt they were a most worthwhile service organization, and therefore became a member.

This began a delightful ten year association that probably taught me more about volunteerism, management, and leadership than any other experience in my life.

On that first night I met many people who I now consider, over 20 years later, to be my good friends.

Two in particular stand out as being most friendly that first evening and through the years I have spent more time with them than anyone else locally.

My assessment until recently was, that though very different in personality, they were equally good friends to me. I loved each deeply and sensed their love returning to me in free-flow fashion.

The past years of stress and health problems in my own life have permitted me to see a major difference in their relationship to me, however, and this new perspective has dictated a variance in how I relate to each of them.

One, when I became ill, made sure she called frequently and stopped by at least once a week for a few minutes. She sent cards, visited in the hospital, brought a Care Bear holding ten balloons (1 for each family member including two dogs and one cat) and a pot of soup for lunch when I returned home. She offered her love, prayers, support and accepting ear as I traversed the mountains and valleys of my journey.

She sensed my needs to not be alone, to be hugged and to be reassured and she filled these needs unsolicited.

While circumstances in her own life became more complicated with the illnesses of husband and parents (plus running a business and managing a younger family) she still made time to be supportive and loving to me.

Certainly she was proving her friendship and love, and I loved her all the more for this.

My other friend, with whom I shared more time and experiences through 22 years, reacted quite differently.

Through four hospital stays she visited once, when my husband called and asked her to stay with me during the critical days after my colostomy for a short period when he needed to run an errand. Through all the months of recuperation before the second surgery she never called, dropped a note or contacted me in any way.

When I could have used her hugs and reassurance most she was no where to be found. When I bumped into her accidentally she was full of reasons why she'd not called — too busy, too rushed, too harried, etc. She also seemed embarrassed and ill at ease.

As I went through illness bouts I found myself saying "she'll come through" just as she had when my husband had experienced his first heart attack some years before.

Unfortunately all of my hopes and expectations led to nothing as my friend became conspicuously absent from my life during the times of my illnesses.

My experience with my two friends has provided great learnings for my life:

First of all, I realize that in the relationship with the second friend, I had been carrying around some hostility ("Why won't she help?!) and a ton of grief at the real loss of what I thought our relationship was: mutually supportive. I have come to the point of accepting my second friend as she is: unable to cope, for whatever reasons, with me in any less-than-strong state. Seeing me vulnerable is simply not something she can handle. Possibly it reminds her of her own vulnerability which is an abhorrent thought to her.

Secondly, I realize that both friends love me, but very differently. One puts me first, the other does not. One responds to my needs, the other her own. It was, I'm sure, equally inconvenient, frightening and sad for each of them to think of me, their on-the-go, in charge, capable friend, reduced to total dependence and needing, yet one put aside her discomfort to be at my side, the other couldn't. And lastly, and possibly most importantly, I came to a peaceful relationship within myself in regard to each. I realize that each of these friends is doing the best she can. Each loves me but demonstrates it differently.

I know that in times of trial and peace, joy and sorrow I can count on one friend to share my journey. The other will only be around when things are going well, when I am healthy and "all-together" and this is valuable information.

Tonic or Toxic?

My grandmother used to call my latter type friend a "fair weather" friend. I think this a very accurate description.

As we look at the relationships we have with others, especially as it relates to our personal dimensions in terms of wellness, I have come to believe deeply in the importance of assessing their true value to us.

Obviously, I can think of no better tonic than the good friends and soul mates of my life. Each brings a special joy, support, warmth, and strength to me in my life's journey. Each is worthy of careful cultivation so that I never take any of them for granted and instead, work lovingly to keep our relationship healthy, balanced, and thriving. They deserve my best efforts!

114

On the other hand, I have had to examine those relationships that were not healthy, balanced or positive. Some I even must label "toxic" rather than tonic, and they deserve only my efforts to terminate them.

Frequently, in talking with others, I hear people hanging on to toxic relationships — with critical friends, disabling co-workers, debilitating clients, and even destructive family members — simply because they think they "should" keep up the relationship even though it is destroying both parties and is draining away positive energy needed elsewhere.

We become ensnarled in negative relationships that bring us little else than sadness, disappointment, and heartache. We constantly put ourselves in line for "one more let down" as we come to expect things from others they simply can not or will not provide, forgetting, of course, that people were not put on his earth to live up to our expectations for them! It is up to us to sort through our relaionships with others to find out which are tonic and which are toxic and relate accordingly to each.

For those that are tonics in our life, I hope we will cultivate them carefully, taking nothing for granted and working hard to keep the relationship growing.

For those that are toxic, I believe we need to carefully assess their toxicity — to see if they are totally so. If so, we need to walk away from them, treating them as a learning experience. Or are they only partially toxic or lacking, so that there are good parts to be salvaged? If so, lets enjoy the parts we can and avoid the parts that bring us sorrow.

I am convinced that how we relate to others and the wisdom we gather in our realistic sorting of our relationships is a most critical part of our over all wellness and health.

When we recognize and accept the fact that people do the best they can and are not put on this earth to live up to our expectations, we can come to peace with them, finding healthy relationships through our perception of them.

I love both my friends. They each love me back. But I have come to accept that they define and demonstrate their love very differently.

One is a friend for all seasons. The other is not, and I am more healthfilled for knowing the difference.

In her wonderfully insightful book, <u>Advice From A Failure</u> Jo Coudert writes: "Friends must be liked at their best, not put in situations in which they appear at a disadvantage. The danger is not so good that you will cease liking a friend who lets you down as that he will cease liking you because he has let you down."[10]

CONCLUSION

The first step in "Taking Care of You" must be a careful assessment of all the dimensions that make up "you."

It is critical that we recognize the many facets and layers that must be in harmony with one another before a balanced wellness can be achieved.

We need to go beyond the traditional four facets of physical, mental, emotional, and spiritual dimensions and examine closely our core dimension of relationships to self and others.

The importance of our relationship to our self, including our self-perceptions, attitudes, curiosity, fitness, growth, and reality, cannot be stressed enough. Equally important is our relationship to others — our faith, our friends, family, co-workers and soul mates — and how we draw the positive relationships closer while ridding ourselves of those that are negative.

When we honestly assess all of our dimensions we have a great part of the necessary information to aide us on our journey to proper care of ourselves — attaining along the way the foundation for good health, happiness, contentment, and grace.

CHAPTER III
END NOTES

1. Coudert, Jo. *Advice From A Failure*. A Scarborough Book, Stein and Day, NY. 1965, p. 100.

2. Pearsall, Paul PhD. *Super Immunity*. McGraw Hill, 1986.

3. Powell, John. *Fully Human, Fully Alive*. Argos Communications, Niles, IL. 1976

4. Ibid. p. 12.

5. Peck, M. Scott. *The Road Less Traveled*. Touchstone Book. Simon and Schuster, NY. p. 308.

6. Coudert, Jo. Advice From A Failure, p. 261. Scarborough Book, 1965.

7. Ibid. p. 257.

8. Ibid. p. 255.

9. Ibid. p. 257.

10. Ibid. pp. 258-259.

CHAPTER IV

GAINING BALANCE

POSITIVE COPING ...

As stress mounts in caregivers there suddenly appear to be an army of advise-givers from family members and friends to doctors and counselors, who glibly entone us to "relax" or "take it easy."

They act as if all we need is a deep breath and a chuckle to relieve our stress. If only it were that simple.

As a young mother with two active sons, I can recall a real sense of anger when my pediatrician told me to "just relax" when the boys both had chicken pox and I'd been up four nights in a row. While managing thousands of volunteer efforts from California to New Jersey under difficult management practices from above, a friend suggested I "take it easy." After my plane had been delayed two hours and I raced to a speaking engagement knowing my audience had been cooling their heels for almost an hour, a bright-faced young man said, "Gee, its a good thing this is so easy for you ... most people would be stressed out!"

Though meant well, each statement showed a total lack of understanding of the amount and intensity of the stressors and what it would really take to relieve them.

As I looked up the word "cope" in the dictionary I found it had several meanings . . . the most frequently used was "to contend with." A second, interestingly enough, was "to cover up."[1]

I will hope that in using coping mechanisms we can learn to contend with and not simply cover up!

In thinking of contending with life I'm also reminded of a tool my husband has in his workshop called a coping saw. I have used it through the years and find it displays all the characteristics a human needs to cope with stress and life in general:

1. It's flexible.
2. It's designed to turn corners and even come full circle.
3. It comes undone at one end so it can fit through a hole.
4. It's very resiliant and cannot be broken easily.

Sounds like just what we need to cope!

Suzanne Kobasa, a health researcher at the University of Chicago[2] has done some studies on coping among executives in high-stress occupations. She noted specific characteristics among those who were healthy, including:

1. A feeling of control over things that mattered to them
2. A greater feeling of involvement in what they were doing
3. A desire to seek challenges, take risks and look for new slants

These executives felt self-reliant, confident and creative. There was a sense of positive personal power that had nothing to do with coersion or dominance (negative definitions of power), and their coping style reflected this positive response to demands. This response choice, or coping, in turn seemed responsible for their good health and balance, lack of buildup of negative stress in their bodies and psyches, and the low degree of burnout.

As we examine coping in general we find a single factor outweighing all others as we move toward managing our stresses. That factor is the feeling of being empowered or in control.

The person who feels empowered still must contend with frustration, anxiety, change, etc. but feels he/she has the next move ... that options and choices are open to them. The successfully coping individual does not feel like a victim of life "but rather has the capacity to be self determining, self-organizing and creative in response to demands.[3]

It is critical to understand that of the coping styles optional to people, several are dysfunctional and negative, others are positive and helpful. It might be useful to look at the options

Dysfunctional Styles:

1. *Withdrawal* — avoiding, fearing or delaying action.
2. *Helplessness* — conviction that nothing you do will make a difference, an extreme form of withdrawal.
3. *Overcontrolling* — trying to be all things to all people; never delegating; trying to dominate everything and everyone.
4. *Internalizing* — keeping feelings buried; trying to meet stress alone.
5. *Emotional outbursts* — the long term outcome of internalizing; feelings build to an explosion point. Normally a shifting of blame (projection) from real source of stress to something safer, ie: anger at spouse is taken out on children or pet, etc.

Helpful, Functional Styles:

1. *Support seeking* — sharing the burden; "the quality and quantity of help we get has been found to be the major determining factor in how well we cope."[4]
2. *Self-renewal* — taking care of the body that has been alerted to respond to stress
3. *Direct action* — problem solving

Please note as you look at these two lists that I am referring to on-going styles or patterns of behavior. There are times when a touch of some of those characteristics found on the dysfunctional list are in fact a helpful strategy. Some control is good, some internalizing can be helpful when sorting through options and even some period of withdrawal to allow yourself a neutral zone. If carried to negative excess or done continually, however, they hurt more than they help.

Common coping strategies used in dealing with job-related stress were listed by Jaffee and Scott in their book From Burnout to Balance[5] and might be a helpful list for you to copy and put up on a bulletin board to remind you of healthy options in dealing with stress:

Most Commonly Used and Effective Coping (ranked in order):

1. Build resistance with a healthy life style.
2. Separate and compartmentalize home and work life.
3. Regular exercise.
4. Talk over problems with co-workers.
5. Withdraw from the situation.
6. Change to engrossing non-work activity.
7. Talk over problem with spouse.
8. Work harder on task.
9. Analyze and change strategy for dealing with problem.
10. Change to different work task.

Coping with the stressors in our life, either at home or at the office, is the necessary groundwork for a healthy existance. With positive coping, comes effectiveness, success and a sense of well being. Without it, comes illness, discouragement and frustration. Whatever positive mechanisms or combinations work for you, be sure to have them at the ready, like a well stocked arsenal of weapons that can fight off the destructive forces of stress and anxiety.

HELPFUL COPING STRATEGIES

The following list of 17 coping techniques and strategies is the list that I have come up with in reading several dozen books, pamphlets, and magazine articles on coping and stress.

You will note, as you read them, a lack of continuity of pattern ... some are "how to" lists, some ask insightful questions of the reader for self exploration, some suggest specific techniques under a particular category, some are simply quick suggestions for coping with specific circumstances, and others are general suggestions in essay format.

All of the categories and most of the specific suggestions have been talked about elsewhere in this book, with many of them foot-noted for deeper exploration by the reader.

Creating a Support System ...

1. Ask for direct help and be receptive when it's offered.
2. List 3-6 people with whom you would like to improve your relationship and 1 action step for each to do so. Then do them!
3. Get rid of toxic relationships.
4. Work on those relationships that are most beneficial. Tell them how much you value them. Don't take anyone for granted.

5. Assess your present network of friends/supporters. Are there weak areas? How could you strengthen them?
6. Keep relationships balanced between giving and receiving, but don't keep score.
7. Choose relationships with people who not only understand you, but understand themselves as well.

Improving Skills for Working with Others ...

1. Clarify joint goals and dreams.
2. Focus on commonalities not differences.
3. Appreciate differences that do exist.
4. Be an active listener ... making contact, clarifying, negotiating options.
5. Work toward harmony.
6. Enable others to be successful.
7. Empower others.
8. Encourage assertion skills.
9. Avoid all personal attacks and aggressions.
10. Keep confidences.
11. Use and encourage helpful humor.
12. Manage conflict positively:
    a. See it as normal and healthy.
    b. Communicate clearly and positively.
    c. Avoid structural barriers and roadblocks.
    d. Work toward shared values where that is necessary to the mission of the work; do not insist on shared values in all aspects of life (ie: religion).
13. Learn how to deal with difficult people (referred to elsewhere as "toads!")

Clarifying Values and Priorities ...

1. List priorities in your life.
2. Rank in order.
3. Determine where you are spending what percent of your time and see if your top priority is getting a major part of your time.
4. Insure that you are a top priority.

Clarifying Needs ...

1. What and who do you need?
2. Which things are you getting/not getting?
3. What action steps can you take to get what you need?
4. Who has what you need? How can you get it from them?

Clarifying Perceptions of Self Esteem ...

1. When do you feel good about yourself?
2. How can you perpetuate such opportunities?
3. Who makes you feel good about yourself?
4. How often are you with them?
   How can you increase time with them?
5. What activities make you feel good about yourself?
6. How often do you get to do these things?
   How can you do them regularly?
7. Where do you feel most valued?
   How often can you be there?

Exploring Self ...

1. When are you aware of your physical, body self?
   What messages come from that part of self?
2. When are you aware of your thinking self?
   What messages come from that part of self?
3. When are you aware of your feeling self?
   What messages come from that part of self?
4. When are you aware of your action self?
   What messages come from that part of self?
5. How do you respond to the message sent by each of these four parts?
6. Are any neglected? Over used? Ignored?

Clarifying Goals ...

1. Where are you now?
2. Where do you want to be?
3. What are your goals for the next year? Five years?
4. What are your lifetime goals?
5. What action steps clarify each goal and make them possible?
6. What choices can you make now to help promote your action steps?

Assessment of Time and Energy Commitments ...

1. Where do you now spend your time and energy?
2. How does this list fit with your goals and priorities?
3. How much time goes for work, play, self, others?
   How does this feel?
4. What steps can you take now to erase any incongruencies between the expenditure of your time and energy and your goals and priorities?

Relaxation Techniques . . . Consider:

1. Rests and diversions (short naps, reading, movie, time with others etc.)
2. Active physical exercise (walking, jogging, swimming etc.)
3. Passive physical relaxation (massage, acupressure, physical manipulation etc.)

Deep Relaxation Technique . . . Consider:

1. Guided imagery
2. Meditation
3. Self hypnosis
4. Biofeedback
5. Stretching and body relaxation

Journaling . . .

1. Keep a daily journal of feelings, events, whatever is important to you.
2. Do not evaluate your writings . . . anything is OK and this isn't a high school term paper to be graded!
3. Note stress points and coping skills
4. Check for progress over time spans

Eating Healthfully . . .

1. Determine the frequency of intake of goods that taken excessively can be harmful: pastries, candies etc; processed meats; canned or processed foods; commercial seasonings; refined sugar; salt; fried foods; alcohol; caffeine drinks; instant breakfasts; cold cereals; quick desserts; beef products.
2. Determine frequency of intake of good foods taken moderately: fresh fruit; fresh or lighty cooked vegetables; water (eight glasses recommended daily); milk, eggs, cheese; flesh food (chicken, fish); whole grains; wheat germ, yeast, protein supplement; herbs; vitamin supplements; balanced meals from different classes of food; snacks of unsalted dried nuts, fruits, or soy beans; fiberous foods.
3. Assess your eating habits . . . do you spend enough time eating? Is it well planned? Is the caloric intake proper? Is it balanced?

Coping With Your Job ... [6]

1. Take charge of your situation.
2. Be realistic about what you can change.
3. Take one step at a time.
4. Be honest with colleagues.
5. Let your employer help.
6. Slow down.
7. Recognize danger signals.
8. Take care of your physical health.
9. Learn to relax.
10. Don't neglect your private life.

Coping With Bereavement ... [7]

1. Be with caring people.
2. Allow time to heal.
3. Express your feelings.
4. Accept a changed life.
5. Reach out for help.
6. Keep in touch with your doctor . . . deal with physical symptoms.
7. Accept reality.
8. Accept that life is for the living.
9. Help others experiencing grief.
10. Don't rush into major life changes.

Coping With Unemployment ... [8]

1. Separate your worth and work in your mind (see section in this book on subject.)
2. Seek help from others . . . friends, professional counselors, loved ones, etc.
3. Stay active and optomistic.
4. Join others in self-help group of unemployed people.
5. Build and maintain a job hunting structure.
6. Avoid blaming.
7. Consider volunteer work to maintain skills.
8. Exercise regularly.
9. Plan low or no cost recreation activities.
10. Consider learning new skills.
11. Be realistic about the timeline to find a new job.
12. Keep up your faith in yourself!
13. Assess strengths and build on them.
14. Brainstorm options freely.

Coping with Everyday problems . . . [9]

1. Accept responsibility for your own life.
2. Try to be objective.
3. Know your own inner resources.
4. Don't try to cope alone.
5. Take a positive approach.
6. Be realistic.
7. Be flexible.
8. Don't strain for absolute control.
9. Take one step at a time.
10. Learn to recognize danger signals.
11. Stay physically healthy.
12. Learn relaxation options for yourself.
13. Laugh!
14. Avoid panic.

Sense of Humor . . .

I can find no stress books that suggest humor as a coping mechanism (though it's mentioned as a valued personality trait in some), but I think it may be a key, under-utilized technique. I'm reminded of Norman Cousin's book <u>Anatomy of an Illness</u>[10] in which he chronicled his active fight against a crippling disease with video tapes of comedies, joke books and having others tell him jokes. He credits his recovery to the use of laughter, and I for one think its a strong weapon, along with faith and companionship, against stress, illness and pain.

I have several friends with whom I laugh a great deal, and I find it helpful to have contact with them when I am under a great deal of stress. Using humor in my presentations delights the audience, but it also is designed to relieve my own tension. Find ways to discover and use humor . . . it truly is the best medicine.

I urge you to look at my coping list as a starting point for your own, so that you might have the necessary tool kit to meet any stressors and changes in your life with a bevy of coping options. I also urge you to read much more about those subjects that pique your interest. For this purpose I have included a reading list of books etc. I have found most useful. Hopefully, you will add to this list from your own experience and explorations. The list is not claiming to be all inclusive, nor is it prioritized in any way. The message it brings is hopefully one of options and choices that are in your control to make as you journey though life.

OPTIONS — HUMANITIES' LIFE SAVERS

Recently I read a report in our local newspaper about a group of 34 nursing home patients. Seventeen of them had come to the home because they had no other option.

The other 17 had looked at several options but had chosen the nursing facility as the best choice.

A year later only one of the 17 who had no options was still alive while 14 of the 17 who chose the facility were living.

Unfortunately, not enough data was given to know health patterns of all 34 (were the 17 "no options" in a desperate health situation, etc.?) yet, I was still impressed by the distinction made between the groups of "options."

I am convinced that we are healthier in all dimensions when we feel we have options in our lives.

Desperation can easily set in, causing mental, emotional, physical, and spiritual stress when we feel we have no choices or options in our life's events.

Frequently I deal with people who seem paralyzed in their actions because they <u>think</u> they have only one, undesirable, choice in some matter.

The most common one organizationally that I run across in my training of volunteer directors is their conviction that a trouble-making, disruptive, energy draining volunteer must be tolerated.

When I point out that as members of the unpaid staff of an organization, volunteers have agreed to certain standards and behaviors, and that therefore there are several options from reassignment to "firing," they are shocked, and often unbelieving!

When in our personal or professional life we think we have no options, we frequently feel "trapped," thus reducing our effectiveness and decision-making abilities. Subsequent or related choices centered on the same subject are often weakened and compound rather than alleviate the problem.

Until Mike Murray made me realize the option I had of leaving an organization that was punishing me for my competencies, I continued to beat my head against a wall.

It really had not occured to me that one option was to go elsewhere, to walk away from disabling management. In case that sounds as if I am a graduate of the "University for the Stupid," let me assure you that my lack of perspective was rather typical of someone in the survival mode.

I was so caught up in trying to circumvent obstacles that I'd lost sight of the fact that another option was to walk away.

I suppose it's like the man who became frustrated in trying to find his way out of a maze made up of two foot hedges. Finally a friend called out to him, "Why not just step over all the rows and get out of there?"

When we begin to identify options that we have — from the sublime to the ridiculous sometimes — we often feel a lessening of tension around an issue.

One of the mental exercises I find most helpful as I am trying to resolve a dilemma is to list all the options I can think of and the consequences of each. I also try to assess the risk, energy, time etc. it will take for each option. When I identify consequences that are negative (what's the worst that could happen?) I ask myself whether or not I could live with this and what I'd have to do to adapt to it.

By going through such an exercise, I find myself realizing there are many options for every circumstance, and I am not locked into any single one. I also have several "Plan Bs" for different options that set the stage for most possibilities.

Leo Buscaglia in his book Living, Loving, and Learning[11] says:

> "I am beginning to believe that maybe the truly mentally
> healthy individual is the one who has the most alterna-
> tives, the most viable alternatives. A person who can say,
> 'If this doesn't happen, what else and what else and what
> else, is possible?'"

Change and circumstance come to us every day. It is up to us to see choices in our reactions to them and to subsequently choose the best options for each. By this feeling of control over one's destiny, we can find greater wholistic health and effectiveness in our life's journey.

AN OPTIONS PARTNER ...

In looking at options, I find it most helpful to call on a close friend or colleague to help me sort out my choices. I find this most valuable when a dramatic change has been imposed on me, and I am going through a period of adjustment or even grief in dealing with the change.

During the first few weeks of adjustment to a colostomy and the possibility of it being permanent rather than temporary, I recognized that my work patterns would need to be altered at the least or dropped all together.

Since training is a primary love and income source, I felt real pressure on my anxiety gauge at what I could do.

Because I had enough sense to realize it was still difficult to think clearly and make good decisions, I turned to Marlene Wilson and Steve McCurley, two close friends and colleagues to have them help me sort through options.

Their perspective and understanding of me and my needs and skills helped reveal options and alternatives I doubt I could have come up with at that stress-laden time.

Many conversations and letters were given over to playing with "what if" possibilities. Not only did they help me draw up an options list, but they also helped me with values clarification and zeroing in on what I wanted to do and could do well.

We discussed a range of possibilities, from simply limiting training dates and writing more books to rehabbing houses and returning to my work as a pen and ink artist. The point was not to make a hard-fast decision at that point (the status of the colostomy or stamina had not been resolved then) but to have a comforting list of options to draw on in any eventuality.

I cannot stress strongly enough the value of having those trusted confidants to help you through those periods when you are seeking options. Frequently their clearer perspective and caring concern can help you expend your horizons and feel supported as you face choices that will impose change and risk.

CREATIVITY — THE FERTILIZER FOR OPTIONS!

Roger von Oech, PhD, has written two of the best books I have ever read on the subject of creative thinking. Their titles give you a glimpse at how he treats the subject: A Whack on the Side of the Head and A Kick in the Seat of the Pants.[12]

In introducing the whole subject of creativity von Oech states: "If you'd like to be more creative, just look at the same thing as everyone else and think something different . . . Creative thinking requires an attitude or outlook which allows you to search for ideas and manipulate your knowledge and experience."

He goes on to share: "You use crazy, foolish, and impractical ideas as stepping stones to practical new ideas. You break the rules occasionally, and hunt for ideas in unusual outside places. In short, by adopting a creative outlook you open yourself up to both new possibilities and to change."

von Oech shares ten things he consider the stumbling blocks to creative thinking. It is important that we identify any such blocks (and others we might impose) as we search for options in our life.

The ten blocks which are considered to be most hazardous to our thinking and my own translations for caregivers, are:

1. "The Right Answer" — Phooey. There isn't just one, singular answer. There's lots — just look around!
2. "That's not logical" — We frequently feel we must use hard, logical thinking to solve problems. This practical, "brass tack" thinking is taught in our schools, leaving us with a belief that it is more valuable than "softer," germinating or free-floating thinking. In creative option seeking, we need to appreciate and exercise our soft thinking ("what would it be like if . . .") and not try to be so "logical."
3. "Follow the Rules" — Fine, as long as they serve the situation. Certainly also, they help keep our society in order, but for creative thinking we need to find ways to challenge rules — to find new solutions and patterns. Flexibility is the order or the day — and that's a rule!
4. "Be Practical" — This is a judgmental phrase of looking at options. Don't be too quick to judge ideas as practical — often the best options result from free-floating, rather impractical germinal ideas we don't immediately squash and brand harshly. Substitute "that's impractical" door-closing statements with "what if" statements that open doors.
5. "Avoid Ambiguity" — In practical situations where ambiguity would cause problems, avoiding it becomes the right choice. However, for creative thinking of options a little ambiguity helps unlock new ideas. Look at something and see what else it might be. Adults look at a hammer and see a tool with which nails can be pounded. A two year old sees a neat thing that smells interesting, can be sat upon, dug with and even tasted! Look for different definitions and perspectives of the same things from various people to stimulate your thinking.
6. "To Err is Wrong" — For option-seeking to be truly creative and exploratory, we need to not be afraid to fail or to risk. When we feel we must not fail we will be reluctant to risk, and if we can't risk we can't really utilize creative thinking. Also there is no such thing as real "failure" if we learn from our mistakes.
7. "Play is Frivolous" — Bah, humbug on this erroneous thought! Playing with ideas is critical to creative thinking. When we play with our options — even if they seem on the surface to be rather ridiculous — we frequently come up with the ah-ha! idea that leads to the best choice.
8. "That's Not My Area" — I learned long ago that I really object to people putting limitations or fences around me. I find some of my best ideas occur to me when I'm nosing around in some unrelated area away fom my concern. The longer I live the more

I'm convinced that we can learn basic solutions in one aspect of life that are applicable in many others. If I did not have the self-permission to explore other "areas," I'd cut myself off from analogous solutions.

9. "Don't Be Foolish" — One of the greatest joys of my life is the fact that I have a number of soul mates who not only accept my foolishness but encourage it! Often while being foolish, I discover "ah-ha! glimpses" at truths that lead me to great solutions and options. A fear of foolishness and a need to "conform" and "be serious" can stifle our creativity more than anything else. Go ahead — be foolish — just choose your timing, location and companions well!

10. "I'm Not Creative" — someone once said: "If you think you can or you think you can't, you're right." The same thing applies to creativity. If you convince yourself you are not creative you'll avoid creative thinking in looking at all of life and its options; you'll shut down your right brain and collect paper filled with "answers" given by others rather than seeking blank paper and a lot of colored pencils with which to draw your own conclusions.

I've given my own interpretations of the ten blocks to creative thinking shared by von Oech in A Whack on the Side of the Head.[13]

Your interpretations might vary just as you might come up with a list of only eight or one of 86⅓. The point is not that we all agree on an exact list, but on the need to remove any blocks that get in our way of creatively identifying options in our life.

There are solutions to all problems.

Or maybe not.

A BETTER WORD FOR "TIME" . . .

"What time is it?"
"Time is growing short."
"How much more time is there?"
"Where did the time go?"
"It's time to get going!"

All of the above are common sayings surrounding time. In this form they each seem to indicate constraint or a dictatorial relationship over us. Several express a feeling of frustration. All seem to say that time controls us, and we are helpless in its grasp.

I have come to believe that a major drain on our wellness is that somehow we have come to an adversarial role with time — seeing it more as an enemy than a friend. This causes us to resent, fight, and even hate time.

If we take a step back from that rather negative perception of time, we begin to realize that by fighting it we are really fighting life.

Because time is life.

Whatever time we have here on this earth, marked for all of us in 60 minute hours and 24 hour days, is actually the gift of life. If we have 80 years or 80 days, this is the time frame of our existence; the canvas on which we paint our experiences, our choices, our life.

As caretakers and helping professionals we tend to use our time in saving others, both in our personal and professional lives. Because we always seem to want to do "more," we often become impatient with the constraints of time, feeling that if we only had more of it, we could do more good, serve more people, accomplish more goals.

The energy drain of such a relationship with time is enormous. I have literally watched people use much of the time they have:

- griping about the fact that here is not enough time to get all the things done that they want/need to do today.

OR

- worrying about not having enough future time to complete a project

OR

- agonizing over the fact that they hadn't been able to do a good job at some point in the past because they had too little time.

If we are to be better stewards of our own resources physically, mentally, emotionally, spiritually and relationally I believe we must write a new definition for time and see it in a new, non-adversarial role.

What if we substituted the word "opportunity" for "time"?

If we saw time as an opportunity for living rather than a constraint, I think we would find greater peace within our self and in our relationship to others and events around us. Certainly we would waste less of it complaining that we have too little of it!

Look what the word — substitute does for our "time" phrases:

"What opportunity is it?"

"Opportunities are growing short."

"How much more opportunity is there?"

"Where did the opportunity go?"

"It's an opportunity to get going!"

Instead of a factor that controls us and provides anxiety, the statements now suggest self-control, challenge and even excitement.

Instead of an adversarial relationship, an explorer, adventurer one is suggested.

Instead of feeling time is a threat or barrier, it becomes a choice and a challenge.

It becomes an opportunity.

Our perception and management of the time/opportunities that frame every moment of our existence, is crucial to our wholistic health. By seeing time in its new, more positive way, we can take advantage of the joys of living now, with less pressure and energy drain given to worrying or even agonizing over time.

Hopefully with this new perspective we can enjoy more of the here and now by smelling the flowers, seeing a beautiful sunset, enjoying the growth of our children at 3 or 33! or any of the other happenings that make up our "NOW." If our attention is focused on time itself rather than on the opportunities it presents in our journey of becoming, we will have lost the art of living in an obsession with its science.

Time is opportunity.

What opportunity is it in your life right now?

EIGHT STRESS REDUCING TECHNIQUES ...

Adult learning consultant Robert A. Jud in the March/April 1985 issue of "The Executive Female" offered eight steps[14] in a stress reducing program that he shares with people across the country, especially as it relates to stress in organizational settings.

I find it interesting to note that we have talked at greater length somewhere in this work about all of them, but it might be helpful, especially for the button-down minds of many left brained readers to share his list here as one technique of stress reduction.

The stress reducers he lists, with my personal elaboration, are:

1. Set Limits ... Admit you can't do it all and plan accordingly! Trying to be all things to all people usually leaves little if any time for you personally and no time at all to smell the flowers. Be realistic so that you can enjoy what you do accomplish and stop flogging yourself for what is beyond you.

2. Time Management ... Apply the techniques of time management to your whole life ... first, determining values and priorities of where and with whom you want to spend your life (and make sure YOU are part of the resultant list!); setting

realistic goals for how you spend your time, and then appropriate pacing, not racing, through your life-plan. Stop making time an adversary; its really a gift and an opportunity when we use it to our advantage ad avoid having it be a stressor.

3. Support Groups . . . You can't have read this far in the book without knowing how much I value and cherish the support people in my life. Make a list of the people and groups you consider your greatest support; then note the opportunities to tap into this support and plan to do so! Avoid being embarassed at having to say "Hey, I need help" . . . this is not an imposition or an unreasonable demand OR a sign of personal weakness . . . it's your way of saying "I trust you" and "I need you," two of the most valued messages true supporters can hear.

4. Personal Empowerment . . . Marlene Wilson, in her book Survi-val Skills for Managers[15] has an excellent chapter on power which goes into detail on the various types of power available to us all. In Jud's article, he focuses on five sources of power:

   a. Reward power — ability to give people something they want . . . money, praise, permission, attention, advancement, affec-tion, etc.

   b. Coercive power — negatively, the power to imperil or threaten; positively, the ability to set limits to help guide and influence, spelling out consequences clearly to affect be-havior.

   c. Legitimate power — power as seen in the eye of the beholder — sharing information that helps others grow; enabling.

   d. Referent power — when you're attached to somebody who has lots of it. Frequently this comes into play when you have a respected mentor or supporters.

   e. Expert power — a major focus of society as it measures com-petencies and expertise; the reason for so much of our present day preoccupation with credentialling; great knowledge as seen by others.

In our culture we frequently only see and use the last type of power, expert, and downplay or even totally discount any of the first four, all of which can be used positively and wisely to feel that we have more control and options in our life.

5. Solving Problems — In studies by psychologist Charles Garfield, he attempted to identify traits of successful people. A key one was that successful people, when they encounter a problem, avoid blaming and move directly to finding solutions, seeing it

135

as a challenge, not an obstacle. Solving problems is the opposite of the panic reaction which leads to high and dangerous stress and deals with options exploration rather than an attitude of "It's all over."

6. Acceptance of Criticism — we need to see criticism as information rather than a personal attack, an indictment or a rejection message. When we categorize it as information we can then make the decision to accept it, reject it, use it, or ignore it and move on wihout feeling stressed out.

7. Develop Flight Mechanisms — I think I might label positive responses more as coping techniques, but whatever you choose to call them these are the ways that you release yourself from the grip of stress — from taking a walk to imagery, deep relaxation or simply a good soak in a hot tub, etc. It's your way of staring stress in the eye and saying, "Sorry fella, you ain't gonna get me, I'll be too busy _____." Fill in the blank by whatever turns you on the most. This is your permission to be self-centered, something rather hard for the helping professional, but necessary to good health!

8. Positive "Head Talks" — giving yourself positive messages rather than terrible ones. We're touching here on self-fulfilling prophesies that we all know can trip us up, and on attitudes that pre-determine everything from success to relationships. Sometimes we create unnecessary stress by envisioning so many worst-possible outcomes that we generate a stress reaction even though nothing is really happening. We need to train ourselves to create up-beat (not Pollyanna, but realistic), positive messages to ourselves, so that we set the stage for success and good endings, not disaster and tragedy. In thinking about going back to work as a trainer after eight months of being "off" while I recuperated, I found it took a lot of self-discipline to convince myself that I could hold up mentally and physiclly to the demands of being on my feet in front of an audience for up to eight hours a day. It was not unusual for scenarios of exhaustion or mental blocks to creep into my thoughts, and I had to work hard to replace these images with ones of a strong Sue Vineyard effectively educating audiences with positive results!

Jud ended his articles by cautioning readers to avoid extremes — a caution I have mentioned before but will reiterate here. I have run into several people who, in the name of stress reduction and "peace," have gone overboard in their techniques, thus <u>adding</u> to their life.

The hysterical jogger, mental imager, religious fanatic, Yoga participant, exerciser, "veggies-and-white-meat-only-thankyou" followers all have missed the point. We are already a too-driven society that lays itself open to attacks by stress, and to add more hysteria to the pattern is rather typical of people who are a few bricks shy of a full load!

Taken with common sense and in proportion to the stress we encounter, these eight steps in tension reduction can help us toward more health-filled and light-hearted days. Taken like cod liver oil — forced down and regimented when the need is not present — it can add to our stress and lessen our life!

FIVE STEPS TO BEING
FULLY ALIVE AND HEALTHFILLED . . .

In August of 1979 a dear friend sent the first of many books to me which we would exchange through the years that we felt were truly helpful to our journey of "becoming."

This particular book, <u>Fully Human, Fully Alive</u> by John Powell[16] helped us discover and frequently discuss our passion for recognizing and using all of the gifts we'd been given so that we could enjoy the fullness of life.

I suppose that each of us too frequently, have encountered people in our travels who, for many reasons, limited the joy of their own (and others) lives because they refused or were fearful of exploring their own depths and plunging ahead in a lifelong learning about themselves and their potential.

I've spoken about attitude enough in this work for the reader to know how highly I regard its importance as a framework through which we view life.

In addition to this all important attitude, there is a logical progression of growth steps as people reach maturity and a point at which they are happy with themselves and in relation to others — a place John Powell would call "fully alive."

As I look again at the issue of being wholistically healthy in all of our dimensions — physically, mentally, emotionally, spiritully and relationally — I am convinced that the basis for this health comes from inner-communication with yourself — a peace, if you will, generated by you (with help from others frequently) for you, and in you.

As I listen to or read ad after ad, article after article on health, I am amused to find so many various remedies or "what ails you" — from stresstabs designed to relieve anxiety to stomach remedies, bran flakes and laxitives that are supposed to take care of our insides. Jogging, aerobics, bounding on a mini-trampoline, jumping rope, and hanging by your heels are all touted as the single activity that will wipe away any problem you might have. Add to these the promise of silver linings if only you'll: eat more fiber, practice yoga, avoid refined sugar, buy a foot massager, eat eight grapefruit daily or phone home, and you have a never ending list of cure-alls for any ill that might beseige any corner of your being.

They each make it seem so simple.

It's not.

When we feel "off-balance" or inharmonious within ourselves, a combination of well-considered stress reducers can aid in recovery of balance and harmony, but will not pull off the whole job without an attitude internally that sets the stage for such recovery.

Wise people have known for centuries that recovery from any ailment comes first and foremost from within. Activities to promote and support such recovery are very beneficial but only in a supportive manner — not as the whole answer to wellness.

In Powell's book,[17] he lays out five essential steps that need to be present to be fully alive/wholistically healthy which I share here, adding my own interpretation for caregivers:

1. To accept oneself. Wholistically healthy people not only accept who they are, but they truly like and love themselves as they are. They feel warm about themselves and enjoy time alone. They are aware of their gifts and their gaps, celebrating the first and forgiving the second. I believe that caregivers who cannot forgive themselves their shortcomings have carved out a difficult path in life for themselves. One stumbling block I see over and over again for those who are dedicated to serving others is an attitude that they must be all things to all people. When they find, naturally, that this is impossible, they brand their "failure" as a personal weakness and frequently become very unforgiving of what they consider a "gap" in themselves.

Powell shares, ". . . a joyful self-acceptance, a good self-image, and a sense of self-celebration are the bedrock beginning of the fountain that rises up into the fullness of life."[18]

2. <u>To be yourself</u>. Have you ever met anyone who you instantly know is trying to be someone they're not? A person at peace with themself and emotionally healthy avoids any such pretend-games and simply is.

In the past two years I've had the uncomfortable experience of having an individual try to be at as many of my training sessions around the country as possible. I know I'm in trouble when I see her ensconced in the front row, taking notes feverishly and responding loudly to every inquiry I make of the audience. At breaks and after the seminar, I know I am in for an oscar performance of who she likes to pretend she is . . . an undiscovered star of the training and volunteer management world. My midwestern/Methodist-Lutheran conservatism has held my tongue so far, but one of these days I'm going to challenge her to be herself so I don't have to put up with the imposter she projects.

It doesn't take a PhD in psychology to recognize that she's afraid to be real and authentic and so she spends her energies trying to be something she's not. I'm convinced that underneath all the bravado and self-promotion is a very nice — though fearful — person, and I wish I could meet her.

Fully alive and healthful people seem to say to the world — "Here's me. What you see is what you get." They do not feel a need to hide behind ego defense mechanisms, and they are not afraid to be vulnerable, thus affording themselves and others a clear view of what is.

Mike Murray, a dear friend and excellent trainer, shared with me the following, which I love:

> "I can be myself or I can be someone I'm not,
>   but I would rather be "me"
> so that those people who love me, love "<u>me</u>"."

I believe that the caregiver who has not only come to terms with themself but has risen above a primary need of approval from others is a healthier, more content human being.

3. <u>To forget oneself</u>. This particular step in becoming fully alive is where I believe most caregivers shine! This is the art of forgetting oneself — the art of loving. "They learn to go out of themselves in genuine caring and concern for others. They are filled with an empathy that enables them to feel deeply and spontaneously with others. They become "persons for others," and there are others so

dear to them that they have personally experienced the "greater love than this sense of commitment," says Powell.

Loving others, Powell points out, is very different from being a "do-gooder." "Do-gooders" he states, "merely use other people as opportunities for practicing their acts of virtue, of which they keep careful count."

Loving others is also much different from "rescuing," whereby a caregiver's real agenda in helping another person is to make the person dependent, thus giving them a sense of power and control and an opportunity to rack up "points" in the Messiah contest. (Beware of falling into the rescuer role unconsciously — it's easy to do when a loved one is floundering, but usually ends up in the rescuers being perceived as a persecuter and finally a victim as described in Marlene Wilson's book Survival Skills for Managers.)[19]

Forgetting oneself and therefore loving others, is a major part of feeling fully human, alive and whole. It is a joy that gives the greatest gift to the giver!

4. To Believe. Powell describes this step in wellness as, ". . . a matter of commitment to a person or a cause in which one can believe and to which one can be dedicated." Caregivers the world over exemplify this commitment as they serve others, a cause or a vision.

One of the greatest joys in my life is the opportunity I have to meet people totally dedicated to various causes and projects — from the election of a particular political candidate, to health care for poverty-stricken children, to cleaning up the environment, to providing quality community theater or hospice health care for the dying. The causes are as varied and diverse as the people, but the single common thread is a selfless, total dedication and commitment to their efforts on behalf of others.

Occasionally, and sadly, I come across someone working in a caregiver role who lacks this commitment, and in such cases, I urge them to leave their position when they can, and strike out on what they can feel passionate about.

I am such a believer that a person really "comes to life," feeling good, healthy, whole and "charged up" when they are doing something passionately. I have urged audiences from coast to coast to find out what turns them on the most and then go for it.

Several years ago Peter Drucker was in Chicago and was asked what was the secret to motivation. His reply paraphrased was: "Motivation heck. Just find out what a person likes to do and is good at and let them do it!" I believe he was speaking of passion and allowing people to pursue those passionate beliefs they have for what the world could be.

"Some people see things as they are and ask why?

I see things as they could be and ask, why not?"

5. To Belong. As the section on relationships will bear out, I believe (passionately!) that we as caregivers need to belong and have a sense of community with others. Soul mates, friends, family, relgious community, fellow workers, colleagues, etc. all offer opportunities to be part of a collection of caring, supportive individuals.

I chuckled when I first heard the "in" phrase of "significant others" but have come to accept it as a label for those who share a caring relationship.

One of my most prized possessions is a Ziggy card sent to me in the hospital and signed by the faculty and staff of the University of Colorado's Volunteer Management Program of which I have been a part since 1978. Its message reads: "Friends are people you like and who like you right back!!!" Messages from many of the people I hold dearest are written all over the back of this stand-up placard and tell me over and over again that I belong to their community; that I am a part of that "family."

A great source of strength for caregivers that I believe is a necessary ingredient to wellness, is the belonging to a community of supportive, accepting, understanding and loving "significant others."

It takes a great deal of effort (and some kissing of toads!) to identify them sometimes, but the effort is well rewarded by the payoff of belonging.

To be able to be what you are, to say even dumb things, to experiment with new thoughts and actions, to be able to laugh and cry and to have others celebrate your successes is pure gold in life, and the stuff of which inner peace, self-acceptance, growth and wellness are made.

Whatever the effort, however long and hard the search, I urge you to find the communities in which you can not only be fully alive, but happily "you" - well, whole and in harmony!

These five progressive steps — to accept oneself, to be oneself, to forget oneself, to believe, and to belong — are part of the package carried internally by a wholistically healthy person. For the person struck down with physical or emotional illness, it can be a support and remedy to aide the greatest surgery or strongest machine.

To be fully human is to be fully alive — healthy in attitude, outlook, spirit, and soul!

CONCLUSION

To be truly healthy in all our dimensions — physical, mental, spiritual, emotional and relational — we need to develop a coping system that is practical, attainable, flexible and adaptable.

We need to look at the options we have and be highly creative as we draw up our list.

We need to develop an attitude toward time that is realistic and positive.

We need to examine stress-reducing techniques and strategies, choosing those that work for us and using them without guilt or question.

As we grow in strength wholistically we need to take the steps that truly make us fully alive, using the gifts God gave us joyfully and effectively.

Certain key stepping stones help us on our path toward realizing our fullest potential and greatest health, and we must keep them clearly in sight in our journey through life:

- Faith in God, self, and others
- Identification of support from others
- An attitude that is positive
  and grace-filled
- A zest for living
- An ability to let go
- A realistic assessment of reality
- A list of options
- A healthy sense of humor!

As we make our way through this thing we call life, we will find sure footing and continued progress when we keep these most valuable stepping stones in focus.

As caring helpers who seek to serve others, we must constantly work to keep ourselves on the pathway to balanced wellness so that our efforts both for others and self are effective and in harmony with one another.

After all, if we don't take care of ourselves, how can we take care of others?

CHAPTER IV
END NOTES

1. Websters Thumbease Dictionary, 1980. Spindex Corp.
2. Jaffee, Dennis and Scott, Cynthia. *From Burnout to Balance,* Mc Graw Hill, NY. 1984.

3. Ibid. p. 99.

4. Ibid. p. 87.

5. Ibid.

6. Coping Series. National Mental Health Series. Washington D.C.

7. Ibid.

8. Ibid.

9. Ibid.

10. Cousins, Norman. *Anatamy of an Illness.* W.W. Norton, NY. 1979.

11. Buscaglia, Leo. *Living Loving and Learning.* Fawcett Columbine, NY. 1982.

12. von Oech, Roger. *A Whack on the Side of the Head, A Kick In the Seat of the Pants.* Harper Row/ Warner Books. 1983/1986.

13. Ibid. *A Whack on the Side of the Head.*

14. Jud, Robert. The Executive Female. Mar/Apr. 1985 "Straight Talk About Stress".

15. Wilson, Marlene. *Survival Skills for Managers.* Volunteer Mgmt. Associates. Boulder, CO. 1981.

16. Powell, John. *Fully Human, Fully Alive.* Argos Communications, Niles, IL. 1976.

17. Ibid.

18. Ibid.

19. Wilson, Marlene. *Survival Skills for Managers.*

EPILOGUE

As the 3½ months following the surgery that created the colostomy went by my tension mounted as to the outcome of the second surgery which was scheduled for October 1986.

The recuperation was slow and painful as the adjustment to a totally new functioning body took form.

I gave a great deal of thought to my life and what had brought me to the operating table. I contemplated the second surgery with increasing concern as I was cautioned over and over by my physicians of the seriousness and complexity of the surgery to close a colostomy and assess further damage done by peritinitus.

On October 14th I entered the hospital for a full and exhausting day of preparation for the operation which was set for the following morning.

After 4½ hours in the operating room and the fine work of two surgeons I emerged with six inches less of my colon but a closed colostomy!

The recuperation of three months was again a slow and gradual one, but the worst was a part of the past.

Each day, with the help of friends and family, I regained strength and renewal and a determination to prevent such stress from building up inside of me again, I did not want to bring about a repeat performance of my hide and seek game with death!

The only question left in my mind was my ability to return to the rigors of traveling and training — being on my feet for up to eight hours a day talking to an audience.

As my first commitment came closer I tried to do everything I could to prepare — going over my presentation, exercising to strengthen my body and legs to the demands of the day, and a great deal of positive thinking about stamina, mental agility, etc.

Two visits (thinly veiled as "co-incidental") by Marlene Wilson and Steve McCurley the week before I was to perform buoyed my confidence and spirits and on February 3, 1987 — one day shy of seven months from the colon rupture — I found myself on a stage in Mobile, Alabama, presenting training in marketing to a room full of volunteer coordinators.

The day went beautifully, the audience was pleased, the coordinator of the event thrilled, and I simply felt good all over, as I believed I'd finally come "home" to where I belonged.

Within three hours of my arrival home the following day Steve and Marlene each called to make sure I was OK and celebrate this victory with me. Within 24 hours I had heard from every one of my support network from Colorado to Virginia who called to share my joy.

In the months that followed I took on more and more work to test what I'd hope would be a return to my training career. With each event, however, I felt an increasing drain on my stamina and reserve.

In May of 1987 I began to revise downward the amount of training I planned to do to try to accommodate my diminished energies. A five day event in August, however, and its resultant exhaustion, caused me to question whether or not I could do any training at all.

Painfully I drew the conclusion that for at least two years I had to set the training segment of my career aside in the hope of regaining my stamina so that I might return to its rigors in 1989. It was a tough decision that underlines the entire message of this book . . . taking care of yourself. I felt as though I could not tell others to care for themselves and then ignore the warnings against my own health and well-being.

My plans for the future are bright, varied and filled with hope, however, as I concentrate on writing, material development and consulting. As I reflect on the events since that hot July night in 1986 in the hospital emergency room I find myself grateful for several things:

First, that I've been given a second chance at life.

Second, that I've been blessed with such wonderfully caring and supportive companions on my journey through life.

Third, that I've had a chance to gain insights that can help not only me but hopefully, through this book and the writing I will do on this subject, others to avoid the stress and life management that brought me close to death in July.

And last, that through all of this I have emerged healthier, happier, more content and whole than ever before.

All in all my life is full and satisfying and whole. I have explored the self that is me, and I like what I've found for the most part, doing repair on those parts slightly out of shape but not unredeemable.

At one critical point following the first surgery, I had to choose life or death.

I chose life.

I'm glad I did.

> "So in the end, it is this that has been said: do not mistake what your lifework is; it is your life. And in that life, all that truly counts is the relationship to the self — the self as deeply as it can be known, as fully as it can be accepted, as genuinely as it can be lived — for from that relationship all else proceeds."
>
> Jo Coudert — Advice from a Failure

Suggested Reading and Bibliography

Anatomy of an Illness, Norman Cousins, 1979. W.W. Norton, NY.

Burnout-The Cost of Caring, Christina Maslach, 1982, Prentice-Hall Englewood Cliffs, NJ.

Christianity and Real Life, William Diehl, 1976, Fortress Press, Philadelphia, PA.

Coping Series, National Mental Health Ass., Alexandria, VA 1986.

Eighth Day of Creation, Elizabeth O'Connor, 1971, Word Books, Waco,TX.

Feelings, Willard Gaylan, MD, 1979, Ballantine Books, NY.

From Burnout to Balance, Dennis Jaffee and Cynthia Scott, 1984 McGraw Hill, NY.

Gifts of Grace, Mary Schram,

Good Grief, Granger Westburg, 1962, Fortress Press, Philadelphia.

How Can I Help?, Ram Dass and Paul Gorman, 1985, Knopf, NY.

I Win, You Win, Ross Van Ness, EdD., 1981, Pendell Publishing, Midland, MI.

A Kick in the Seat of the Pants, Roger von Oech, PhD., 1986 Harper Row, NY.

Life After Stress, Martin S. Hafer, PhD., 1983, Contemporary Books, Chicago, IL.

Living, Loving, and Learning, Leo Buscaglia, PhD., 1982, Fawcett Columbine, NY.

Love, Medicine and Miracles, Bernie Siegel, MD. Harper Row, NY. 1986.

The Precious Present, Spencer Johnson, MD, 1981, Doubleday, Garden City, NY.

The Road Less Traveled, M. Scott Peck, MD, 1978, Touchstone Books, NY.

Stress, Sanity and Survival, Robert Woolfolk, PhD. & Frank Richardson, PhD, Signet Books, NY 1978.

Stress Without Distress, Hans Selye, 1974, Signet Books, NY.

Success is the Quality of Your Journey, Jennifer James, PhD., 1983, New Market Press, NY.

Super Immunity, Paul Pearsall, 1986. McGraw Hill, NY.

Survival Skills for Managers, Marlene Wilson, 1981, Volunteer Management Associates, Boulder, CO.

Transitions, William Bridges, 1980, Addison Wesley Publishing, Reading, MA.

A Whack on the Side of the Head, Roger von Oech, PhD. 1983, Warner Books, NY.

When Bad Things Happen to Good People, Harold Kushner, 1981, Avon Books, NY.